Love Your Scar

Love Your Scar
Breast Cancer

Adrianna Holman
RSHom, BSc NutrMed

www.loveyourscar.com

www.homeopath.moonfruit.com

Copyright © Adrianna Holman 2010

Part of the *Love Your Whole Self Series*

A Great Granny Smith Publication

ISBN 978-1-4461-7022-9

All rights reserved. No part of this publication may be reproduced or distributed in any form without the prior permission of the author and/or publisher.

The author is not a medical doctor and the content in this book is for information purposes and in no manner replaces the relationship with your primary physician or medical team. You should inform your medical doctor of any supplements, exercises and/or remedies you choose to use. The reader assumes all responsibility for following any of the information within.

North American spelling is used intentionally.

Cover design by Carolyn Baltas
Back cover photo by Lisa Noel Greenfield
Illustrations by Ali Crossman
Publishing assistance by Tony Loton

Contents

Contents	1
Acknowledgements	7
Note from the author	8
About the author	9
Introduction	11
Daily self-care	13
Daily Care Plan	14
SECTION I: Foundations of Healing – The Why	15
Understand your scar	17
WHAT IS A SCAR?	17
3 HEALING STAGES OF WOUNDS	18
TYPES OF SCAR	19
ADHESIONS	20
FASCIA	21
Different surgeries	25
BREAST SURGERIES	26
RECONSTRUCTIVE SURGERY	28
COMPLICATIONS	32
AFTER SURGERY	34
OVER TO YOU	36
Your lymphatic system	37
WHAT DOES LYMPH DO?	40

WHY IS THE LYMPH SYSTEM SO IMPORTANT?	41
THE SPLEEN	42
WHITE BLOOD CELLS AND THE LYMPH SYSTEM	42

SECTION II: Help Yourself Heal – The How   43

First basic exercise post-operation: 45

RHYTHMIC DEEP BREATHING	46
MANUAL DRAINAGE OF LYMPH FLUID	47
WALKING	48
DRY SKIN BRUSHING	49
DRY SKIN BRUSHING ROUTINE	50
ACTIVATE YOUR LYMPH	51
TRAMPOLINE OR REBOUNDER	52

13 Lymph Activation Exercises   54

KEEP A RECORD	54
STARTING OFF	55
Exercise 1: Rock the boat	*56*
Exercise 2: Frog's legs	*57*
Exercise 3: Twister	*59*
Exercise 4: Backstroke	*60*
Exercise 5: Cat stretch	*61*
Exercise 6: Child's pose	*62*
Exercise 7: Seaweed	*63*
Exercise 8: Seated Twist	*64*
Exercise 9: Neck rolls	*65*
Exercise 10: Scratch your back	*66*
Exercise 11: Opera singer	*67*
Exercise 12: Doorframe stretch	*68*
Exercise 13: Spider up the wall	*69*

Massage therapy — 70
- CHEST DRAINING MASSAGE — 71
- RELIEVING BREAST CONGESTION — 72
- PROFESSIONAL MASSAGE — 73

Scar massage — 74
- INTRODUCTION — 74
- SELF-ADMINISTERED MASSAGE – OVER TO YOU — 75
- HOW SOON SHOULD YOU BEGIN SCAR MASSAGE? — 76
- UNDERSTAND YOUR START POINT — 77
- PREPARE YOUR MIND — 78
- GETTING STARTED — 79
- GOING DEEPER — 80

Natural beauty alternatives — 83
- AVOID PARAFFIN OR MINERAL OIL — 84
- ANNETTE'S FAVORITES — 86
- CLINICAL TRIALS OF VARIOUS PLANT OILS — 86
- SKIN DEEP TOXICITY RATING OF NATURAL PRODUCTS — 89
- INLIGHT ORGANIC SKIN CARE — 90
- INLIGHT OFFER AND CHARITABLE DONATION — 93
- DR HAUSCHKA — 94
- AMANDA'S RECOMMENDED DR.HAUSCHKA PRODUCTS — 95
- NEAL'S YARD REMEDIES — 96
- TRILOGY — 97
- WELEDA — 98
- SKIN BLOSSOM — 99
- NELSONS SCAR CREAM — 99

Nutrition — 101
- WE'VE NEVER HAD IT SO GOOD? — 101

AVOID TRANS FATS!	105
ORGANIC FOOD	107
EAT MORE FRESH FOOD	113
LOAD UP WITH VITAMIN C	114
FOODS HIGH IN VITAMIN C	115
SUPER GREENS	116
ANTIOXIDANTS	117
STAR-PERFORMER ANTIOXIDANTS	118
OMEGA 3 FOODS	119
GENERAL FOOD GROUPS	120
LIQUIDS	123
YES PLEASE:	128
LESS OF THESE:	129
HEALING DIET MEAL SUGGESTIONS	130
Breakfast:	*130*
Lunch/Dinner:	*131*
Pudding:	*132*
Super snack:	*133*
SUPPLEMENTS	135
FOODSTATE NUTRIENTS	137
Pre-operative supplementation	*138*
Immediately after surgery	*139*
Long term supplementation	*140*
EXTRA DIETARY SUPPORT	141
DIET AND CANCER: CLINICALLY SUMMARIZED	143
Homeopathy	**144**
Bach Flower Remedies	**149**
Metaphysical Healing	**152**

BURNING LETTERS	154
HEALING VISUALIZATION	156
CHAKRA HEALING	159

Conclusion   163
CONTACT ADRIANNA	165

Resources   167
PEOPLE	167
Scar Massage Therapists	*167*
Integrated Medicine Physician	*167*
Breast Consultants	*167*
PRODUCTS: SKIN CARE	169
PRODUCTS: HOMEOPATHIC AND BACH FLOWER REMEDIES	170
PRODUCTS: NUTRITIONAL SUPPLEMENTS	171
PRODUCTS: FOOD	171

Appendix: Different Surgeries   173
RECONSTRUCTIVE SURGERY	174

INLIGHT Organic Line Softener voucher   179

Acknowledgements

This book is dedicated to the patients at London Bridge Hospital for whom I have provided advice on post-operative scar and lymph care since 2002. They repeatedly requested I write it down so, thanks to their encouragement, here it is.

My gratitude goes to London Bridge Hospital, especially Gill Welch and Jane Loughnane, for appreciating the value of complementary therapy and integrating it into the Oncology department. I feel very fortunate to work with such caring professionals as Nicole, Barbara and Kelly (to mention but a few).

My heartfelt thanks to my editor Eleanor Jacques who took a manuscript and helped me make a book.

My love goes to my colleagues Amanda Berlyn and Annette Dawson for their trust in me and their dedication to our patients.

Lastly I express deepest thanks my husband Mark for his steadfast love, encouragement, support and sense of humor that lifts me time and again.

Note from the author

This book is a guide for those who are currently managing or have had breast cancer, their carers and loved ones as well as therapists interested in working in this area.

The information provided is an adjunct to the treatment you are receiving from your primary physician and in no manner substitutes such care. Do seek professional help if necessary as the advice herein is presented at a broad level rather than specific to the individual.

My aim is to empower patients and encourage active participation in the healing process. There are two main sections: the 'why' and the 'how'. Use what appeals to you at this moment and try new techniques as you advance in your healing.

Holistic health involves the mind, body and soul of a person. All three levels must be engaged to experience true vitality. We are all works in progress and the ability to flow through the challenges of life allows us to grow.

I wish you the very best in your journey.

About the author

Adrianna Holman has been in the healing profession since 1992. After completing her Bachelor of Science in Business Administration (BSBA) from the University of Denver she managed a health store in the US while studying massage therapy at the Health Enrichment Center under Sandy Fritz. In 1998 she moved to London to study homeopathy full time at the College of Homoeopathy, gaining her registered status with The Society of Homeopaths at the end of the three years. Further studies include homeopathic focus in toxicology, homeopathic methodology and understanding cancer, a foundation course in Kinesiology and a variety of techniques for rebalancing the energy systems of the body with Delphi University. She recently completed her Bachelor of Science focused on Nutritional Medicine with Thames Valley University.

In 2002 Adrianna initiated complementary therapy at the Oncology department of London Bridge Hospital and is currently the lead practitioner for the Complementary Therapies team providing support for cancer patients and staff. Adrianna is also one of the original practitioners at Nelsons Homeopathic Pharmacy Clinic, the pharmacy itself being the oldest in Europe. She was a founding practitioner and Head of Homeopathy at The Third Space Medicine. In addition to her work in the UK, Adrianna treats patients worldwide via telephone consultations and has a private practice in Bermuda where she grew up and still has family ties.

Introduction

Breast cancer is on the rise. More than a million women worldwide are diagnosed every single year. In the US the Center for Disease Control and Prevention supplies the statistic of 191,410 women diagnosed in 2006. The charity Breast Cancer UK reports that in the UK incidence of breast cancer rose by more than 50% in the last 25 years, and it is now cited as the country's most common cancer in women under the age of 35. In 2005 more than 45,500 British women were diagnosed with breast cancer, or about 125 women every day, and the lifetime risk of developing breast cancer was projected 1 in 9 in 2001. Of the total breast cancer cases that do occur in the UK less than 10% can be attributed to a hereditary link. This means that as many as 90% of all breast cancer cases result from other causes.[1]

Having seen firsthand what my patients go through this is an overwhelming set of statistics. However, I have also witnessed how the same patients get through the trauma of their diagnosis, surgery, radiotherapy, chemotherapy, and out the other side, and I have been privileged to play a part in their recuperation and healing.

Recovery from breast cancer surgery involves many levels of repair. The first step is to acknowledge and face your new condition. Over the years I have been touched to the core by the grace, dignity and incredible strength of the women I have worked with.

---

[1] Breast Cancer UK website www.breastcanceruk.org.uk/statistics

Love Your Scar

My objective in writing this book is to encapsulate my knowledge and experience of working with these women during their breast cancer recovery, and to share our collective experiences to the benefit of all women embarking upon the same difficult journey.

I am also determined to change the stigma surrounding scars. Too many women come into my treatment room and immediately apologize for the appearance of their scars. They are embarrassed by something over which they had no control. They feel disassociated from their scar and see it as a constant symbol of the disease that led to it and of their own fear.

I want to encourage you to take a different view. Your scar is a sign of your strength. It is a testimony to your body's ability to heal and overcome surgery, chemotherapy, radiotherapy and all the other trials you have undergone, physical and emotional. It is nothing to be ashamed of: you are here and life is beautiful.

Daily self-care

Your daily self-care may look like a huge to-do list that you can't possibly fit in around your busy life. Here's the thing though: if you are reading this you have most likely had surgery for a life-threatening disease. It's time for you to re-evaluate who and what gets a piece of you every day.

Is there anything (or anyone) that drains your energy? Do you need to let go of some relationships or change the parameters of others? Perhaps it's time your family pitches in more. If you say things like "Never mind, I'll do it", the people around you will tend to back off and let you. It is important that you allow them to help however they can.

Instead of feeling guilty about it ask yourself if anything else *really takes priority* over you getting yourself well. You don't need extra time, just a shift in your priorities. Stop worrying about things that do not really matter in the long run. Mum, wife, CEO – it's time to put yourself first.

The following Daily Care Plan is merely a suggestion for putting together the entire 'How to' of the book. Do what you like. At the very least I recommend you do the scar massage and the Lymph Exercises that are pertinent to the location of your scar.

Daily Care Plan

In the morning, after waking

- drink hot water with ¼ fresh lemon
- five to ten minutes of rebounding
- dry skin brush before bathing
- after bathing lymph clearing exercise
- scar massage apply nourishing oils to scar
- breakfast and supplements

During the day

- deep breathing exercise
- green smoothie
- healing visualization
- energy remedies in water - Homeopathy or Bach Flower remedy

In the evening

- five to ten minutes of rebounding
- lymph exercises

Before bed

- healing visualization
- scar massage
- chakra healing

SECTION I: Foundations of Healing – The Why

Understand your scar

What is a scar?

Human beings are quite remarkable healing machines. Our bodies naturally attempt to heal whenever and however damaged. Trauma to the skin causes new fibers - scar tissue - to be generated to fix the damage. Because it needs to be very versatile scar tissue does not have the ability to replicate the original tissue; instead it knits the broken or wounded areas together with a one-size-fits-all tissue, creating a physically distinct repair site, or scar.

Scars come in all shapes and sizes depending on the type of wound or surgery, age of the patient, site of the injury, general nutrition, and patient's own individual genetics and healing capabilities. An associated infection with a wound can alter the size of a scar, as can repeat surgeries in the same area. Internal injuries such as deep bruising can trigger a scar response as these damaged tissues also have to mend.

3 healing stages of wounds

1. The Inflammatory Stage starts with the initial infliction of the injury and lasts for a few days. With any inflammation there is redness, heat and swelling as blood vessels constrict to control bleeding; platelets and thromboplastin form a clot; specialized white blood cells clean the wound of bacteria; and various chemical substances are released to begin the healing process.

2. The Proliferative Stage lasts about three weeks, but can take longer depending on the severity of the wound and whether or not infection is present. In this stage a matrix of new skin cells and blood vessels form. Specialized cells called fibroblasts generate collagen to fill the wound, making a framework on which the new tissues build. Capillaries - tiny blood vessels - supply the new cells with nutrients and oxygen and support collagen production. (Collagen is the main component of the final scar.) The increased blood supply gives the wound its pink color which fades in time.

3. The Remodeling Stage begins 2-3 weeks after the initial wound and **can last up to two years**. Collagen continues to form, becoming more organized to increase the robustness of the resultant tissue. During this stage the density of the blood vessels diminishes and the wound gradually loses its pink color. The shape of the wound may change as the collagen restructures and once complete the area will have 70-80% of the strength of the original tissue. Quite amazing!

Types of scar

Contrary to popular belief, not all scars are the same despite all being formed of the same scar tissue and subject to the 3 stages of healing outlined previously. In fact, there are three types of scars: atrophic, hypertrophic and keloidal. **Atrophic scars** are depressed and cause an indentation in the skin. Examples are acne and chicken pox scars. Surgical scars are mostly **hypertrophic scars** which are elevated initially and subside over time becoming flatter and paler. **Keloid scars** are actually non-malignant tumors formed by scar tissue that continues to grow beyond the boundaries of the original incision or injury. Most breast surgery will result in hypertrophic scars.

The limitations of scar tissue make scars delicate and less resistant to ultraviolet radiation, so it is important to protect them when out in strong sun. Scars lack sweat glands and hair follicles which can make them troublesome if they cover a large area as part of the functioning aspects of skin will be lost. The greater the area of scarring from your surgery the more rigorous you will need to be with massage and stretching.

Adhesions

Imagine your scar as a boat in a choppy harbor, with people throwing off ropes in different directions in an attempt to keep it steady. Adhesions are like these ropes.

Adhesions are fibrous bands of scar tissue that extend beyond/behind an injury and which bind together parts of the body which would normally remain separate. They are a natural response to injury whether by infection, trauma, surgery or radiation and they are the body's attempt to repair and restore stability.

It may also surprise you to discover how far the adhesions can travel from the original wound. Posture can be greatly affected if adhesions form on the ribs pulling the chest inwards. After a few sessions of scar release you will notice an increase in range of motion and a return to a more normal, comfortable posture.

To help understand how adhesions and scars affect more than just the wound area let's have a deeper look at one of the main ways the body is held together: the fascia.

Fascia

Fascia (pronounced *fash-ya'* in this context) is strong connective tissue and literally wraps around everything in our bodies. You can visualize fascia as a long sheet of plastic wrap or cling film weaving its way throughout the body.

Fascia thickness ranges from sheer and delicate to substantial and very strong bands such as found on the outer leg. Fascia surrounds and isolates the muscles, forms the foundation for cartilage and bones, is vital to nerves, blood and lymph vessels and provides structure and protection for the internal organs.

It forms a continuous vast supporting network from head to toe. Tendons that attach muscle to bone, and joint capsules and ligaments which attach bone to bone are all fascia. If you eat chicken, next time you cook one have a look at the flat, white tendon that is often attached to the breast. When you pull on it there is often a thin, tough sheet of tissue attached. That is fascia.

Tight fascia can form rigid knots or undesirable connective adhesions, causing pain in the body. These are the trigger points your massage therapist finds and releases in a deep massage. If someone is offering a myofascial release massage, this is the freeing of the fascia too tightly bound to the muscles. It holds imprints of our old injuries and poor postural habits and therefore dictates how much freedom of movement we have.

Fascia exists in three distinct levels/layers[2]. Subserous fascia, the layer around the organs, can also form knots and adhesions and these can become painful and restrict the organs from functioning optimally. **All nerves and blood vessels run through the fascia,** so a tight area of fascia will result in poor nutrient exchange to the surrounding tissues. As a result metabolic wastes build up and aggravate the pain receptors, causing further pain.

To illustrate how fascia relates to a scar, grab a handful of your shirt at the front of the shoulder and see how it pulls the rest of the garment from the surrounding areas. Where you are grabbing can be likened to a scar. The creases radiating from the bunched-up area are the adhesions; the pulling sensation is the restrictive fascia. This pulling has to be released to restore proper mobility through the body.

If a nerve within its tight casing of fascia becomes adhered to a nearby muscle, bone, skin or blood vessel then the nerve will be irritated when the muscle is moved. This can cause tingling, burning, numbness or weakness in the area.

Remember that everything in your body is connected via fascia, so blood or lymph restrictions caused by restricted fascia can lead to edema,

---

[2] Superficial fascia lies directly under the skin, serving as a strong layer of connective tissue between the skin and the underlying muscles. The second level/layer is the stronger and denser deep fascia which covers the muscles and keeps them divided and protected. Finally, subserous fascia lies between the deep fascia and the major organs of the body. Subserous fascia is more flexible and leaves space for the organs in the body to move freely.

Understand Your Scar

swelling and temperature changes. This is why scar release techniques are so important to the healing process.

When one of my patients, Faye, first came to see me she was wheelchair-bound due to her inability to breathe properly. Her surgery had taken place six years earlier. I placed my hand above her navel and asked her to breathe into that space, i.e. the bottom third of her chest. I observed her chest rise at the top, completely skip the middle and slightly raise the very bottom. She was panting from the exertion of trying to take a single deep breath. Her scars felt like tight bands around her ribcage and they were severely restricting her ability to inflate her lungs.

> *CASE STUDY: Adhesions preventing recovery*
>
> ## *Faye's story*
>
> *"I started chemotherapy in September 2009 having been diagnosed with secondary breast cancer. A month into chemo I began to have problems with my breathing. I couldn't walk more than twenty yards without becoming breathless, almost to the point of collapse. My breathing pattern was totally erratic.*
>
> *I was sent for a heart and lung scan, but the scan came back normal. I then saw Adrianna who, after listening to my troubles, asked if she could work on my scar. She commenced deep tissue massage and I noticed an improvement after the first half-hour treatment. After the second treatment the improvement in my breathing was dramatic and I could now inhale and exhale fully."*

Faye had suffered needlessly. In her case the adhesions ran from her breast scars all the way to the bottom of the ribs and the entire area was compressed.

I followed up with her a few months after the two short scar massage sessions and her breathing continues to be healthy and normal. She has had some restrictions in different areas, meaning the fascia is releasing and changing with new areas needing to be addressed. Now she is equipped with the knowledge of how to administer self-massage she is managing these herself. Faye still continues treatments with me but more on a maintenance basis.

Different surgeries

Where your breast cancer is and what type of surgery you have will mostly determine the location and length of your breast scar. It will also have great bearing on the way your fascia is affected which in turn can change your posture.

If you have reconstructive surgery using tissue from another part of the body, whether the back, abdomen or buttocks, you will have to invest more time and energy into your healing as you have more area to cover.

With more intensive surgery it will take longer to restore flexibility and mobility. It is not impossible – just more involved.

For therapists and those interested, a more detailed description of the surgeries is in the Appendix.

Breast surgeries

Lumpectomy

In a lumpectomy the scar is usually quite small and sometimes there may be a small dent in the breast. The amount of tissue removed varies greatly from person to person. This is the least invasive surgery and therefore causes minimal impact on the tissues.

Approximately 1 in 8 (12.5%) of women will need to have a second operation to remove more tissue if on examination of the lump there is indication that pre-cancerous cells are still in the breast.

If further surgery is required there will be additional scar tissue in the area.

Segmental excision (quandantectomy)

This is similar to a lumpectomy but more tissue is removed from the surrounding area.

Mastectomy

- A simple mastectomy removes only breast tissue. The lymph nodes and muscles are unaffected.
- A simple mastectomy **and** sentinel node biopsy or node sampling removes the breast tissue and the lower lymph glands situated within the armpit.

Different surgeries

- A modified radical mastectomy (also called a total mastectomy and axillary clearance) removes all the breast tissue and all of the lymph nodes in the armpit.
- A radical mastectomy removes all breast tissue, all lymph nodes in the armpit and the muscles behind the breast tissue. This is only done if the cancer is found in the chest muscles under the breast.

Mastectomy scars usually run in a line across the chest from the breastbone to the armpit. When there are breathing difficulties, especially in double mastectomies, it is crucial to check the scars for adhesions. Full range of motion may also be compromised in the shoulders and neck so look for adhesions anchoring up as well as down.

A note about lymph

When lymph nodes are removed there is a greater chance of lymphedema or swelling in the arm on the side of surgery. The more lymph nodes taken from the breast area, the more the other areas of lymph concentration in the body will need to be given attention.

Varying degrees of lymph glands are removed in:

- *the simple mastectomy and sentinel node biopsy*
- *a modified radical mastectomy*
- *a radical mastectomy*

The importance of the lymphatic system is explained in its own section.

Reconstructive surgery

Reconstruction after a mastectomy may take place at the same time as a mastectomy or your surgeon may wish to wait, possibly up to a year, before performing reconstructive surgery. It is important to discuss this fully with your surgeon. Breast reconstruction either uses an implant of some kind, in which case the scar will be localized to just the breast, or there are 'tissue flap' reconstructions which involve other parts of the body.

Every woman is an individual and scars pull the fascia in different ways depending on how you have healed as well as any previous postural habits. These descriptions are based on the most common patterns I have seen with my patients.

The illustration shows the most common scar positioning for the various types of reconstructive surgery.

Different surgeries

Most common scar positioning for reconstructive surgery

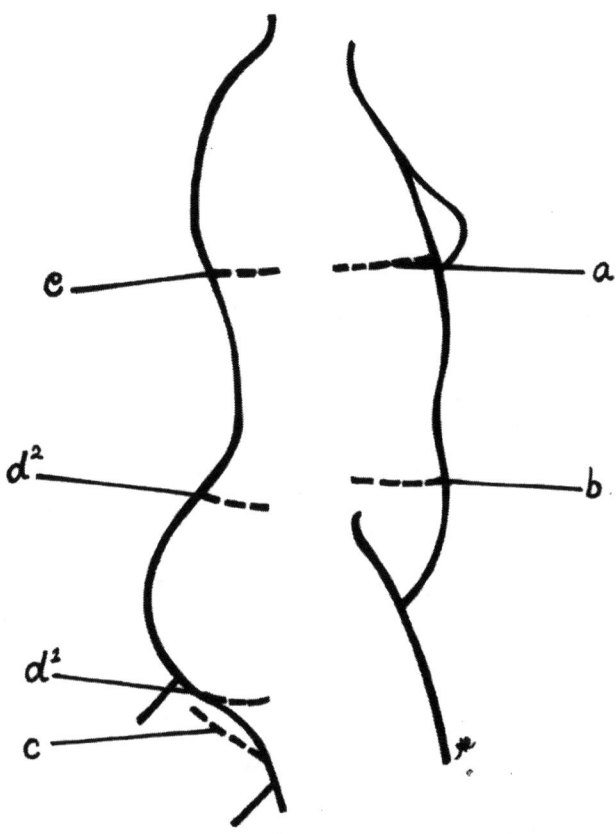

a: Mastectomy scar
b: TRAM flap and DIEP flap reconstruction
c: Free TUG flap reconstruction
d[1]: IGAP (Gluteal flap) reconstruction
d[2]: SGAP (Gluteal flap) reconstruction
e: Latissimus dorsi (Lat flap) reconstruction

(b) TRAM flap reconstruction

This surgery uses the abdominal muscle (transverse rectus abdominis muscle) and moves it into position to reconstruct the breast. The scar involves an oval shape around the breast, a long scar across the lower abdomen and sometimes the belly-button is reconstructed. Two scars on the front of the body are likely to pull towards each other. This may affect posture in that it feels difficult to stand up straight. Additionally the lower back may feel tight. Work on the scars first to see if this releases the lower back.

If you have a TRAM flap surgery my suggestion is that **when you are ready** you make sure to stretch the front of the body regularly. You can lie back over a Swiss ball or stretch back over the back of a sturdy chair or sofa. The twisting exercises in the Lymph activating exercises will also be of great benefit. Please double check with your surgeon that this is suitable for you (especially if you have mesh inserted) and go slowly!

(b) DIEP (deep inferior epigastric perforator) flap reconstruction

This surgery is almost identical to a TRAM surgery but no abdominal muscle is taken. This entails microsurgery and takes much longer to perform. The scars will be the same as for a TRAM: an oval shape around the reconstructed breast and a scar along the abdomen above the pubic line. Do the same exercises as for a TRAM reconstruction.

Different surgeries

(c) Free TUG flap Reconstruction

This is a relatively new operation suitable for slim women with small breasts. This procedure uses tissue from the upper inner thigh, namely the gracilis muscle. The scar is at the top of the leg and there can sometimes be a problem with fluid building up in the wound area on the leg. Be certain to ask your surgeon about the safety of doing leg exercises, particularly "frog legs" in the Lymph Activation exercises.

Adhesions here are more likely to create problems in the hip or pelvis. Gently stretch the groin muscles and inner thighs once you are able in order to keep fluidity in the hip joint.

(d) Gluteal flap reconstruction

This surgery uses skin and fat, and sometimes muscle, from the upper or lower buttock. It is usually performed when abdominal tissue is unavailable due to previous surgeries or when the woman is very slim.

The scars for a Gluteal Flap depend on the type. An IGAP (d^1) surgery results in a scar hidden in the buttock crease whereas a SGAP (d^2) surgery results in a scar that is higher up on the buttock. In a Gluteal Flap reconstruction the breast scar is oval. Look for the potential of restrictions in the hip and lower back. I have also found the hamstrings can become very tight on the side with the scar. There may also be an over reliance on the opposite leg so both sides can be tight: one side from the surgery and the other from doing all the work. Check both.

(e) <u>Latissimus Dorsi (lat flap or Muscle Pedicle Flap) reconstruction</u>

This surgery uses muscle and skin from the upper back. An oval section of the Latissimus dorsi muscle is used to create the new breast. The scar around the reconstructed breast is oval and the scar on the back is usually horizontal along the bra line. There may be a pulling sensation around the side of the body between the two scars or some women have a sensation of tightness inside the body between the front and the back. Neck and shoulder tightness can be a problem as well as the potential for overuse of the back muscles on the other side.

Complications

Sometimes surgeries do not go according to plan, even under the most ideal conditions. We may not heal well, stitches may not hold, drains and wounds can get infected, as well as our bodies simply not coping well with the trauma. These incidences can lead to a more complicated scar pattern in the body.

We cannot see the underlying stabilizers the body has put into motion after surgery but we can feel them. If you are at all unsure or confused about what is happening with your scars it is best to see an experienced massage therapist who can help you understand how your body is reacting to the surgery or surgeries.

Different surgeries

CASE STUDY: More complicated scarring pattern

Sue's story

"I was diagnosed with breast cancer in April 2009. As is always the case with this diagnosis the doctors move fast and you are required to take some really big decisions. Given the size of my cancer I elected to have a mastectomy together with reconstructive surgery using my own tissue.

The SGAP flap operation had a 98% success rate and seemed like a really good option. The danger of statistics... I happened to be in the other 2% and had a really fraught time including four days in intensive care, four operations and six blood transfusions. To think it was the chemotherapy I was most worried about! So I was left with no reconstructed breast and massive scarring to my breast area, a huge scar on my buttock where the donor tissue had been taken and a graft site on my thigh to repair the skin that was taken.

It was going to take a lot of work to heal from the operation and get full mobility back in my arm, shoulder and buttock. Being a sport and fitness person this was really important to me.

Fortunately I met Adrianna and she has taken 'holistic' to a whole new level. She has given me homeopathic advice, massage, deep scar massage and has been a great listener. I feel very fortunate to have met her and question where I would be on my rehabilitation without her skill. It is a highly personal thing showing your surgical scars and allowing someone to touch them. Adrianna's skill in scar healing and the benefits I gained from her understanding of this area were phenomenal."

Love Your Scar

After Surgery

Following your surgery you will return home with aftercare instructions from your hospital. Check with your surgeon, but from what I understand there is no need to disturb the dressings for the first five days or until your first follow up appointment.

The best way to have a healthy scar is to do everything possible to reduce the risk of infection. Eat a very nutritious diet, rest, rest, rest and drink plenty of water.

The reason I emphasize rest is because we do so much healing when we sleep. Your body repairs on a nightly basis and when recovering from surgery you may feel exceptionally tired. Please do not soldier through trying to recover in one week. Take naps if you are tired and let people 'do' for you.

As you will be told, if you experience any of the following after your surgery telephone your doctor immediately: unusual pain, swelling, heat around the wound, extreme tenderness, any oozing discharge, any bad smell or if you become dizzy. Keep the area dry and do not touch it. If your wound becomes infected you will probably be given antibiotics and further wound care instruction.

<u>Bra or no bra?</u>

Please do what your surgeons tell you to do! If you are told to wear a support bra all the time, wear it all the time. Mr. Nicolas Beechey-

Different surgeries

Newman[3] of The Harley Street Breast Clinic and London Bridge Hospital explains why:

> *"With fuller breasts it may be suggested to wear a bra in the day, night and even in the shower for support. If you do not you can place too much pressure on the wound and it will not heal optimally. On the other hand, while most breast scars are rounded, some are straight or 'radial' and if these scars shorten it can be a problem. For radial scars it is better to <u>not</u> wear a bra and let gravity keep the scar stretched by the weight of the breast to limit distortion of the scar".*

If a breast with a radial scar were held up in a bra the scar would heal shorter causing future complications and require considerably more massage. Follow your surgeon's advice to the letter to give yourself the best start in the long term care of your scar.

Manuka honey

Manuka honey is rapidly gaining a reputation in mainstream medicine as a topical application for healing infected wounds[4]. In one study radiation-

---

[3] See Resources – People

[4] The healing qualities of Manuka honey come from the antibacterial properties of its key ingredient MGO or methylglyoxal, formed as a side product of several metabolic pathways. MGO exists in other foods, but in nowhere near the same level/concentration as Manuka honey. Put some in your tea as well for extra benefit.

induced wounds responded well to Manuka honey dressings, with marked improvements in the size and condition of the wound area as well as a reduction in pain. No adverse side effects were noted.[5]

Surgeons at The London Bridge Hospital recognize its value in combating wound infection. Mr. Beechey-Newman recommends use of Manuka honey on dressings when the wound shows signs of infection. Ideally infections would be avoided but if it happens, ask your surgeon about using Manuka honey to help.

Over to you

With your surgery complete and you back at home the healing process commences. Up until now you have been largely in the hands of healthcare professionals. This is when you start to participate actively in your healing. Make no mistake; you have a critical role to play in the rate and quality of your recovery.

In order to gain the most benefit from the exercises and techniques described later on it is important that you have an understanding of what you are achieving by using them.

The next section covers the lymphatic system. Even if you have not had lymph nodes removed I would advise you to read through in order to understand and appreciate your body's incredible healing mechanics.

---

[5] Robson V, Cooper R., 2009. Using leptospermum honey to manage wounds impaired by radiotherapy: a case series. *Ostomy Wound Management,* 55(1):38-47

Your lymphatic system

The lymphatic system consists of lymph (a fluid), lymph vessels (the tubes along which the lymph travels), lymph nodes (small round organs), bone marrow, diffuse lymphoid tissue such as the tonsils, and lymph organs such as the spleen and the thymus.

The lymph system is a point of interchange with the blood.

Your blood carries oxygen and nutrients to the tissues and removes toxins and carbon dioxide. The smallest blood vessels are called capillaries and from them the lymph and blood escape into the surrounding tissue.

Lymph, also known as plasma, is a non-cellular fluid that goes where the blood cannot. It carries nutrients to feed the tissues and also contains white blood cells called lymphocytes that help protect the body from infection.

If you have lymph nodes removed from the breast area as part of your surgery, the lymph flows to the nearest concentration of lymph nodes to be processed. Therefore it is imperative to keep the other nodes working optimally particularly in the groin. You should actively support this through the lymphatic draining exercises in Section II.

The Lymphatic System

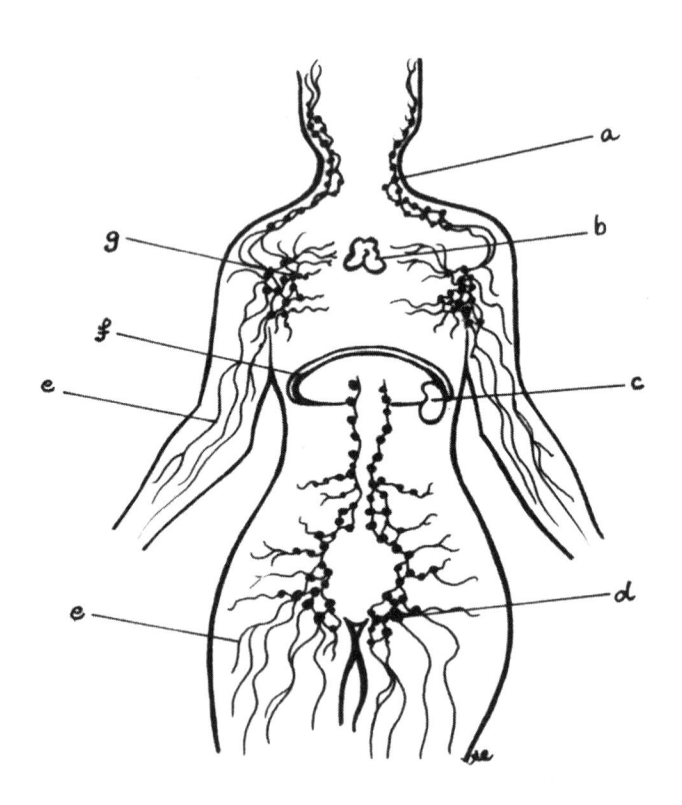

a: cervical lymph nodes
b: thymus gland
c: spleen
d: inguinal lymph nodes
e: lymph vessels
f: diaphragm
g: axillary lymph nodes

Your Lymphatic System

You may be surprised to learn that the volume of lymph in the body is about double that of blood. There are also roughly twice as many lymph vessels as there are blood vessels, so it is a significant body system.

The vast network of lymph vessels **flow against gravity** towards the central lymph glands located in various parts of the body, mainly in the groin, stomach, breastbone and armpits.

Backflow is prevented by single direction flap valves in the lymph vessels. Unlike the circulatory system that has the heart pump the blood, the lymphatic system has no pump and relies instead on muscular contraction (i.e. movement and exercise) to move the fluid around the body.

Lymph passes through vessels of increasing size and several lymph nodes before returning to the blood. It does so through the two main lymphatic ducts, the Right Lymphatic Duct and the Thoracic Duct, both of which are located at the collarbones.[6]

---

[6] The Right duct drains lymph from the right side of the head, neck, right arm, right lung, right side of the heart and the upper surface of the liver (right side of the ribcage, or thorax, and its contents). The Thoracic duct receives the lymph from the rest of the body including the entire left side and both legs.

What does lymph do?

One of the easiest ways to visualize the working of the lymph is to compare it to your local rubbish collection service. It generally runs smoothly: the trucks come regularly and gather up the bags, tins, boxes and other bits and take them away to be sorted and disposed of at a central processing plant. If the roads are well maintained and nothing gets in the way, it all happens swiftly and efficiently.

Imagine that the street is in disrepair and the trucks cannot move as quickly. Getting the rubbish off the street takes longer and it begins to decompose in the sun. This is what happens when we do not exercise or drink enough water, or eat foods that clog the system such as hydrogenated fats, excess sugar and general junk. The whole body becomes sluggish and the lymph struggles to remove wastes effectively.

Now suppose some of the trucks are permanently taken off the road. This is what happens when lymph nodes are removed in surgery. How many depends on the surgery and will determine how much extra support you need to give your lymph system to ensure all your body's waste products are still being collected.

You now require a different strategy to remove the rubbish with fewer trucks. It is critical that you keep the roads clear and in good repair to facilitate the efficiency of the trucks you still have. Stimulating the areas of high lymph node concentration will help the body stay on top of waste removal.

Why is the lymph system so important?

- Tissue drainage: every day around 21 liters of plasma fluid carrying dissolved substances escape from the arterial end of the blood capillaries and into the tissues. Most of this fluid is returned directly to the bloodstream, but 3 to 4 liters of fluid are drained away by the lymphatic vessels.

- Absorption in the small intestine: fat and fat-soluble materials such as vitamins are absorbed into the lymphatic vessels of the *villi* – small hair-like projections on the inner wall of the small intestine, which increase the total surface area.

- Maintenance of the immune system: the lymphatic organs are responsible for the production and maturation of lymphocytes, the white blood cells primarily responsible for immunity. Bone marrow also produces lymphocytes and is considered lymphatic tissue.

The spleen

The spleen and thymus gland are organs of the immune system with high levels of lymph activity. Exercises in Section II will assist these organs in flushing the lymph and compensating for any nodes lost in surgery.

The spleen is our largest lymph organ and highly active in the body's defense. Abnormal and old red blood cells are destroyed in the spleen and the breakdown products sent to the liver. Unlike the lymph nodes the spleen is not entered by any lymphatic vessels, protecting it from diseases carried by the lymph to the nodes for destruction.

White blood cells and the lymph system

Lymph plays a vital role in protecting the body from foreign materials known collectively as antigens.[7] The immune system response to the presence of these is to dispatch cells called phagocytes via the lymph system. These cells act like a 'Pac-man', engulfing and trapping the antigens, and releasing them when they come into contact with the white blood cells designed to destroy them.

Having surgery for breast cancer does not automatically mean full lymph removal. However, if lymph nodes *are* removed in surgery it is helpful to understand how significantly this will affect your body and why you need to support this vital system.

---

[7] Including abnormal cells, pollen, bacteria, fungi and larger molecule drugs

SECTION II: Help Yourself Heal – The How

First basic exercise post-operation:

It is time to reorganize your life around your new self-care regime. It's important to make this a priority.

BreastCancerCare.com states that obesity increases the risk for all types of estrogen receptor-positive breast cancers. Women who gain weight after menopause are most at risk because estrogen is produced in fat tissue and high amounts of fat increase the level of estrogen in the body, thereby leading to faster growth of hormonally sensitive cancers.

The good news is that losing weight after menopause is likely to decrease the risk of breast cancer, a view endorsed by Dr. Mark Harries, a breast consultant at The London Bridge Hospital.[8] This suggests that staying slim is a good prevention against breast cancer. It is important to make exercise a part of your daily routine if it isn't already. Besides, exercise is more fun and far more beneficial than strict dieting.

---

[8] See Resources – People

Rhythmic deep breathing

Deep breathing will instantly relax you while refreshing the body with oxygen. It can be done anywhere and at any time, especially before visualization or meditation, or if you ever feel yourself tensing up from anxiety or when emotionally overwhelmed.

Sit comfortably with your feet flat on the floor, or lie down. Exhale fully, open your mouth and sigh out loud saying 'ahhhh'. When you think all the air is gone, give one more little puff of an exhale and feel your stomach pulling back towards your spine.

Inhale slowly through the nose down to your stomach. Relax your stomach muscles and let your belly push out.

Take a full breath to a count of four, filling the abdomen first and finishing in your upper lungs. Your shoulders may rise slightly. Hold your breath for a count of two, then reverse and exhale for a count of four, letting the air leave the lungs from the top to the bottom. As you finish breathing out feel your belly pull in. Pause here for a count of two.

Repeat at least seven times or for five minutes.

Basic exercise

Manual drainage of lymph fluid

Your post-operative body will have swelling, redness and tenderness. Once the bandages are removed and the wound is healed you can assist your immune system by boosting the lymph with the following simple technique. (My tip is to incorporate this when toweling off from your bath or shower):

- Take long slow breaths into the abdomen.

- Press gently and rhythmically on one side of your breastbone up towards your shoulder using the flat of your opposite hand.

- Repeat five times each side. Be gentle and allow a pause between each press. This helps to cleanse the area and relieve congestion.

Your ability to move will be restricted for some time after surgery. Do the lymph presses and deep breathing as well as any physiotherapy exercises you have been given. Be extra aware of your posture and keep a straight spine - your natural urge will be to protect of your injury and to curl your body inwards to avoid bumping the area. Start doing the exercises more vigorously when you feel stronger and your wound is completely healed.

Walking

Walking is simple, free and a slow pace is perfectly fine when recovering from surgery. You want to move your body to help move wastes out of the cells and increase circulation for both the blood and the lymph.

Ideally an hour of exercise a day will keep you in great form. Work up to it. Don't stress if all you can manage is ten minutes. Keep building up your stamina by increasing the amount you do by a couple of minutes a day.

I am fully aware that chemotherapy can knock the stuffing out of you. If all you can handle is the deep breathing exercise, the manual drainage and the Frog's Legs lymph exercise (mentioned shortly) you will still be doing your body good.

Another way to move the lymph without moving your body is with dry skin brushing, explained next.

Be consistent, be patient and be kind to yourself. You will get there.

Basic exercise

Dry Skin Brushing

As you now know, the lymph has its own system just beneath the skin, running alongside the circulatory (blood) system. Skin brushing is extremely beneficial as it moves the lymph while also removing dead skin cells allowing your skin to breathe. After doing this for some time you will have smooth velvety skin.

Use a natural bristle brush[9] with a long handle- **dry** - on your dry skin before bathing, (washing it in a mild soap at least once a week). Avoid going directly over any fresh scars or skin complaints such as eczema.

Always move the brush in slow gentle strokes towards the heart. You want to push the lymph towards the areas that have high lymph node concentration, mostly found in the trunk of the body. Avoid fresh scars, sensitive or sore skin. Make the strokes long and sweeping. Once your skin is used to it you can use a bit more pressure. A minimum of three strokes per section is recommended.

---

[9] Available from health stores and many local pharmacies. Make sure it is natural bristle. There are also more specialty circular lymph brushes that have rubber nodules amongst the bristles to help move the lymph along.

Dry skin brushing routine

Start at the bottom of your feet and in long strokes brush up the lower leg to the knee.

Go from knee to the groin on the front of the thighs, then up the back and over the buttocks, sweeping round to the front top of the thigh ending in the groin where there is a high concentration of lymph nodes. You are literally pushing the lymph fluid into the nodes for processing.

Breathe!

Continue up the lower back taking time to go over the kidneys and go as high as you can reach. For the front of the body, circle around your belly-button clockwise three times. Brush up the front of the torso to the heart.

Now, move to your upper body: start with one hand in the air and brush from the hand to the shoulder. When you get to the armpit, be gentle as the skin is delicate. Brush the back of your neck, down your shoulders, and down your upper back around to the armpit. Brush gently across the chest from the armpit to the breastbone, taking deep breaths all along.

Basic exercise

Activate your lymph

To recap, your lymphatic system has no heart to pump it, and flows largely upwards and against gravity. To do this it depends on muscular contractions. Post-surgery it is therefore essential to regain an active lifestyle as soon as you are able to help your body pick up and dispose of the rubbish.

In addition to general activity, (and/or to compensate for more limited activity as an immediate consequence of your operation) you should add some or all of the following specific exercises designed to stimulate the other areas of high lymph node concentration and maximize lymphatic flow.

Adjust them to suit your body and your needs. The key is regular exercise, with emphasis on regular.

Trampoline or Rebounder

One of the best exercises for the lymph is rebounding (bouncing) on a mini-trampoline. Remember, lymph works against gravity, so every time you bounce you give the lymph a great flush. This exercise dramatically boosts circulation while still being gentle on the joints. If there is any pain in the wound area, stop! Wait until the scar has fully healed.

Adding in arm movements will enhance the effect; even simply holding them above your head while bouncing makes your body work harder. Try rebounding both with shoes and without to see which you prefer. You do not need to lift off the rebounder and bounce to the ceiling to gain benefits - even moderate bouncing is very effective.

The benefits of rebounding include a reduction in stress and tension (it's really fun), an improvement in circulation, an increase in heart and lung capacity, improved co-ordination and balance, and most of all it is excellent for boosting the lymph system and therefore the immune system —all this with no jarring the joints.

If stability is a concern there are rebounders with attachable bars you can hold while you bounce. There is a wide range of rebounders on the market from high street brands to more expensive ones. I would recommend you start with one from the high street (it might squeak and the mat may not be very bouncy) but you will see if it is something you think you will stick with. If you like it and you feel the benefit; it is worth investing in a top quality one.

Basic exercise

Bouncing little and often will bring more benefits than one long session. Two to three 10-minute sessions per day on the rebounder will be enough to activate the lymphatic system.

Have a quick bounce while the kettle is boiling, during your favorite TV show or first thing in the morning to wake up your system. You will get an energy boost as more oxygen is fired around the body when you exercise. Breathe deeply and fully throughout.

There are online 'classes' and resources for rebounding exercise routines. Have a look to see how creative you can be while bouncing. The next section outlines thirteen different exercises designed to activate the lymph.

13 Lymph Activation Exercises

If you are uncertain about the suitability of any of these exercises taking your personal case into consideration, please check with your doctor or nurse before starting. If in doubt leave it out.

If you have recently had surgery, do what you can and ease off if you experience pain. Some exercises will be harder than others. Take your time – persistence is the key. If you don't have time to do all these exercises together, divide them into 2 groups and do the lying-down ones before you go to sleep.

There are **13 lymph activation exercises** in all, some of which may replicate exercises you have been given by your breast care nurse or physiotherapist. Start gently and keep a record of your progress.

Keep a record

Keeping a journal of your progress can be a great motivator. As you note your improvement you can see how far you have come in your recovery. So many women find this empowering as the small daily efforts pay off BIG TIME when you have your full range of motion back. Please trust me when I say you do not want a restriction if at all possible as this reminds you of what you can't do. I want to help you to get on with your life. These exercises will reward you with better posture and freedom of movement, not to mention a sense of purpose and peace with your progress.

Lymph activation exercises

Starting off

Start by lying on the floor or bed. Bend your knees and place your feet flat on the floor, knees pointing upwards. Gently massage the lymph nodes in the groin just to wake the area up. Take some deep breaths and move the diaphragm muscles in the abdomen. Really push out your lower stomach with each breath and think of a happy Buddha with a plump round belly, relaxing the abdomen completely. Let your breathing return to normal, still inhaling slowly and deeply. With the actual exercises do not do the Buddha belly – instead you need to stabilize the center of your body. Before you begin each exercise, make a quick check that your core muscles are steady.

LOCK YOUR CORE

Exhale and imagine your belly button sinking backwards into the floor, (visualize a string pulling your belly button towards your back) and then hold the muscles firmly in this position. Your breathing is now located more in the ribs so you can visualize the ribcage expanding sideways in order to keep your core locked.

If you have troubles, find a Pilates teacher to help you.

Love Your Scar

Exercise 1: Rock the boat

This is a very small movement which helps to warm up your coccyx or tailbone. It also awakens your core and pelvic muscles which you will need throughout these exercises.

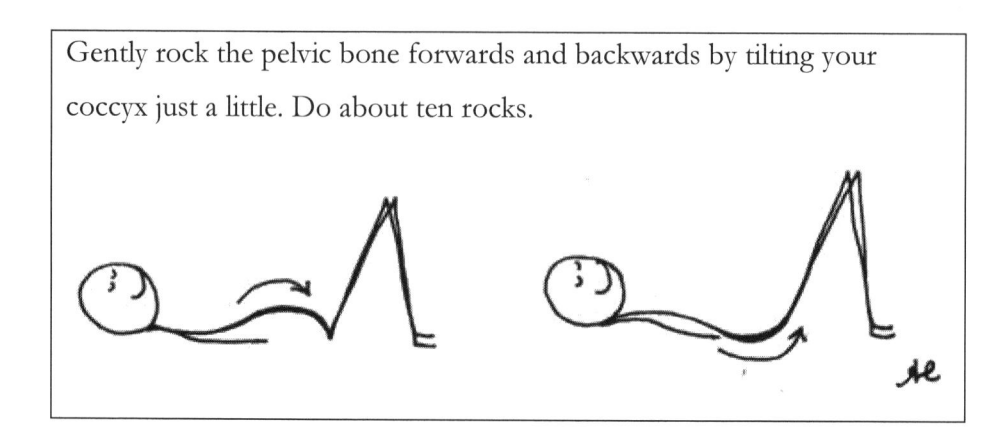

Gently rock the pelvic bone forwards and backwards by tilting your coccyx just a little. Do about ten rocks.

Then move onto…

Lymph activation exercises

Exercise 2: Frog's legs

The lymph node area in the groin is a large one. If you have had lymph nodes removed from one or both armpits you need to work the ones in your legs even more. This exercise stimulates the lymph in several ways.

Firstly, your feet are in the air using gravity to drain lymph into the lymph nodes in the groin, the deep breathing helps flush the lymph and pumping the leg muscles helps accelerate the flow of lymph.

Lie on your back with your legs in the air. If you are too tired to do the exercise simply rest your legs and feet up the wall and breathe deeply into the abdomen. This still helps the lymph tremendously.

Rotate each foot a few times in each direction and point and flex the feet. Take a couple of deep breaths and get ready to love your lymph! Lock your core again and start:

Love Your Scar

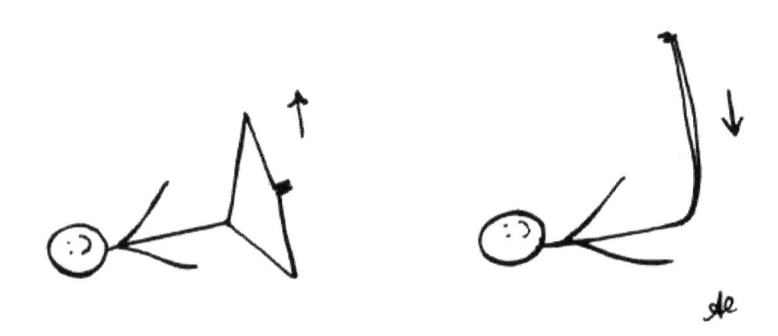

Bend your knees outwards keeping your feet together at the soles to make frog's legs, and slowly pump your legs up and down. If you like you can place your hands under your lower back for more support.

Keep breathing, inhaling as you bend the legs and exhaling as you straighten them. Try to do at least ten repetitions to start with and build up to a couple of minutes as you become stronger over time. Keep your core strong and move slowly.

A modification is to place both legs up the wall and keeping the core tight, bend one leg in towards the body at a time. Breathe deeply throughout.

Lymph activation exercises

Exercise 3: Twister

Twister massages the internal organs and can help move the bowels. The whole torso is stretched which helps mobility throughout. If you have had abdominal surgery, take this one very slowly.

Stay lying on your back and put your feet back flat on the floor keeping your knees pointing up. Extend your arms comfortably to the sides and steady yourself with your hands palms down. Take a deep breath in and, as you exhale, gently allow both bent legs to fall to one side. Keep your shoulders in contact with the floor if possible, palms facing down. Let your head fall gently in the opposite direction to your knees.

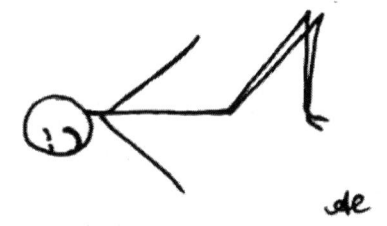

Feel the stretch in your ribcage, lower back, arms and neck. Take a few deep breaths, continuing to stretch into the pose on each exhalation. Slowly change sides, remembering to *activate your core muscles* before you do so. Place a pillow under your knees for support if needed.

Take another couple of breaths on the other side and move on to…

Love Your Scar

Exercise 4: Backstroke

Backstroke is a very controlled movement and you may have limited range of motion after surgery. Just keep practicing and the tissues will start to ease. This helps stretch the chest, arms and shoulders while activating the lymph nodes in the neck, arms and chest.

> Start with your knees bent upwards and feet flat on the floor, arms straight by your sides. Bring one arm slowly over your head and extend it as far back as you are able. Then reverse the move, lifting your arm upwards and back over your shoulder, returning it to the start position. As you do so, start lifting the opposite arm upwards in the reverse move. Repeat five times either side.
>
> Remember to keep your tummy engaged - imagine anchoring it to the floor - and prevent your hips and feet from rocking. Keep breathing deeply and establish a rhythm.

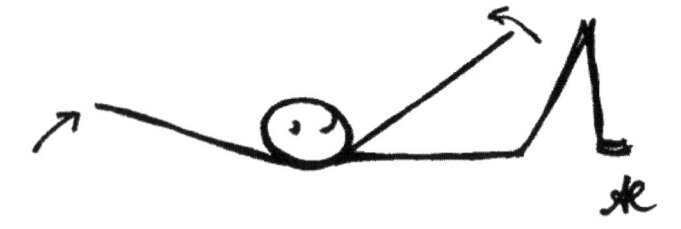

Lymph activation exercises

Exercise 5: Cat stretch

*The Cat Stretch is lovely for the whole spine as well as the internal organs. It stretches out the front of the body from the chin to the pelvis as well as the back from the top of the head to the tailbone. Use the breath with this exercise to massage the internal organs. When you exhale pull the tummy muscles up slightly. As before, if you have had abdominal surgery, **do not** exaggerate the movement. Go only as far as you can.*

Roll over onto your side and push yourself up onto your hands and knees. Look up, breathe in and arch your back, moving your tummy towards the floor taking the spine into a 'U' shape. On the exhalation curl over making a rainbow out of your spine, and push all the air out of the lungs. Go very slowly.

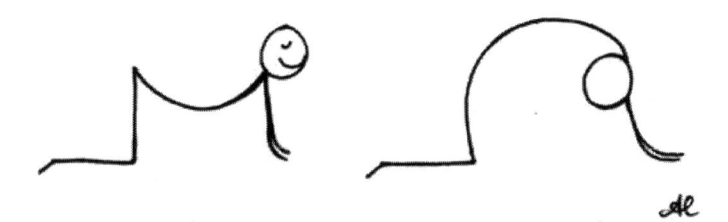

Repeat three to five times.

Exercise 6: Child's pose

In yoga this is a calming pose. Close your eyes, let your face fully relax, feel your forehead soften completely. This stretch is so good for the arms, back and shoulders and will be of particular benefit in cases of cording. To me this is a posture of surrender and serenity. Use it whenever you have some quiet time to yourself.

Sit on your heels with your hands on your knees. Stretch your arms out in front of you while keeping your buttocks on your heels. Let your fingers gradually creep forward. Rest your forehead on the floor if possible and if not use a pillow to support your face so you can relax.

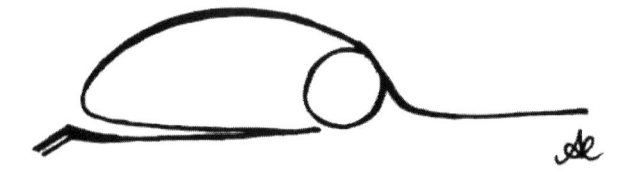

Take ten long slow breaths, exhaling fully with a sigh, letting all the tension leave your body with this pose.

Move into a comfortable sitting position, ideally cross legged, for the next set of exercises. Sitting with your tailbone on a small cushion allows your knees to relax more. You can also put pillows under each knee for full support.

Lymph activation exercises

Exercise 7: Seaweed

As it sounds, this is a gentle flowing movement to help open the sides of the body from the armpit to the hip as well as the small muscles between the ribs. The arms also receive a lovely stretch.

Put your right hand out next to your body and lean over to the right with your left arm over your head, trying to keep both buttocks on the floor. Slowly and gracefully change sides, moving your arms through the air as if they were sprays of seaweed rolling gently on the waves.

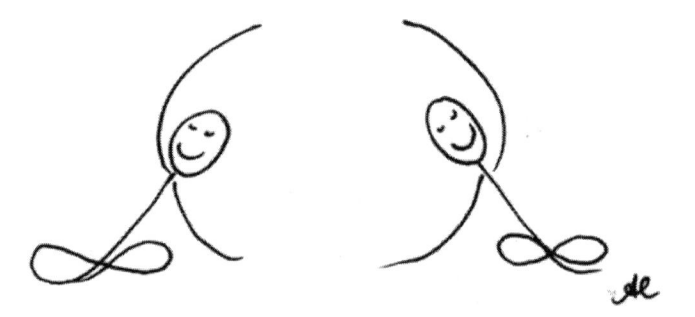

Repeat for a total of 10 times, five each side. If lateral movements are difficult, do what you can and watch for progress.

Exercise 8: Seated Twist

The seated twist is similar to the lying Twister. It has a different action on the hips and groin because of the seated position. It helps squeeze the internal organs gently, improving digestion and elimination while freeing possible rib adhesions. As with Twister, go gently if you have had abdominal surgery.

While sitting in a cross-legged position twist your whole torso gently to the left placing your left hand on the floor directly behind your spine. Place your right hand on your left knee to help hold the position and gently turn your head to look over your left shoulder, stretching the neck. Take two deep breaths, return to center and twist to the right, right hand behind the spine, left hand on the right knee, looking over the right shoulder. Take two refreshing breaths and return to center. Repeat.

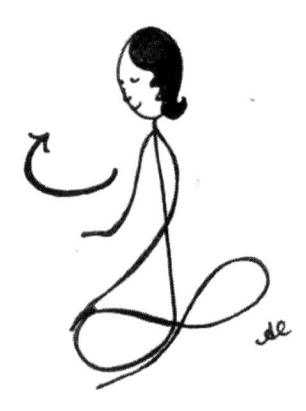

Lymph activation exercises

Exercise 9: Neck rolls

Stretching the neck helps activate the lymph nodes situated along the collarbone. It relieves the tension so commonly held in the shoulders and releases possible restrictions in the chest and front neck muscles.

Roll your shoulders back, straighten your spine and actually sit on your hands, palms up, so you are grabbing your bum. Your shoulders should be anchored down by the position of your hands. Allow your head to drop gently forward and let it roll slightly from side to side, just a little to start with. Roll your head to the right so that your ear is over your shoulder and take a couple of breaths. Do not roll backwards! This is a side to side only rolling through the front.

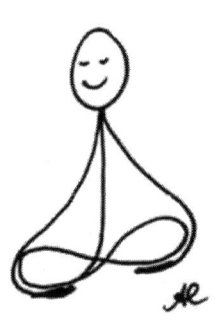

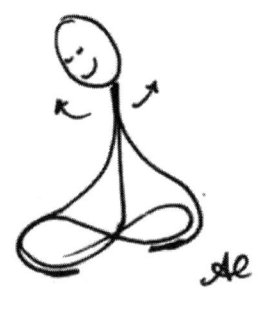

Try not to let your shoulders creep up. Keep them down and rolled back so the neck receives the full benefit of the stretch. Roll to each side three or five times depending on how tight it feels.

Love Your Scar

Exercise 10: Scratch your back

This exercise helps to open up the chest and shoulders while stretching the top triceps muscle, and is a great one to help with cording - do what you can.

> Holding a belt or dishcloth in your left hand, raise your left arm over your head, bend at the elbow and reach your hand down (still holding the belt) as though to scratch between your shoulder blades. Twist the other arm up behind the back as though scratching the middle of your back. Grab the belt or cloth dangling with your right hand. Gently and slowly pull the top arm down, breathe, and then slowly and gently pull the bottom arm up.
>
> Do this in little movements and eventually your hands will meet in the middle. When you are as far along on the belt as you can be take two deep breaths. Gently release the belt and do the other side. You will undoubtedly find one side is easier than the other.

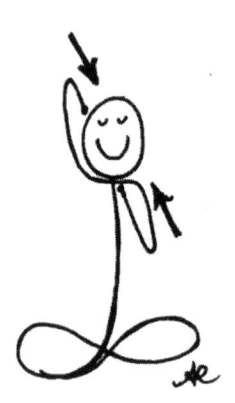

Lymph activation exercises

Exercise 11: Opera singer

This simple exercise helps mobility in your ribs and armpits and improves lymphatic flow through the torso. Moving the arms in opposite directions from each other gives a diagonal stretch to the chest and ribs.

Stand up and stretch one arm away from you and to the side, looking at your hand as though you were on stage singing your heart out. Move the other one down and away in the opposite direction.

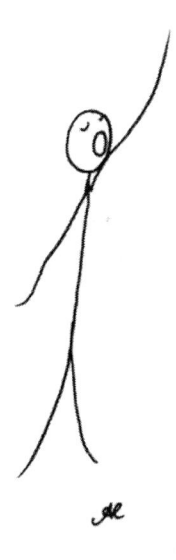

Change sides a few times and feel the mobility in your ribs and armpits. Take deep breaths to help stretch out the ribs and enhance the lymphatic flow. If you feel moved to hit a high note, do!

Exercise 12: Doorframe stretch

This exercise stretches the chest. After breast surgery there can be a tendency to very naturally and instinctively roll in the shoulders to protect the scar. This can lead to restrictions in the chest though so gently puffing out your chest using the doorway as a stabilizer keeps the front of the body stretched.

> Choose a suitable doorway and place your arms on the door frame at chest height. Take a very small step forward and feel the pull in your chest and shoulder muscles.
>
> If this feels okay, take another very small step forward. Take a full breath, stretch out the ribcage and relax. This is a subtle stretch, not very big and can be done surreptitiously without anyone really knowing what you're up to.

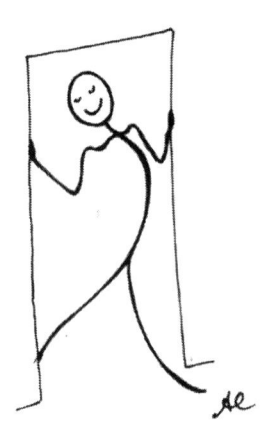

Lymph activation exercises

Exercise 13: Spider up the wall

This exercise is a very common one given post operatively by physiotherapists and breast nurses. Crawl the spider (your fingers) up the wall and allow all the small muscles in the arm, chest and shoulder to gently open up and release.

Face the wall and stretch one hand up placing it on the wall in front of you as high as you are able.

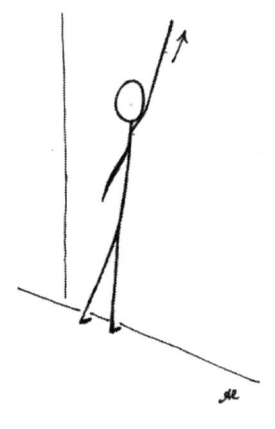

Creep your fingers higher and higher up the wall feeling the stretch in the chest and arm.

Doing these exercises regularly will move along swiftly in your recovery. Remember to keep track of your progress for motivation.

Massage therapy

Massage has so many amazing benefits. I think the most important is the fact that you are touched. You may feel your scar is alien or something to be avoided and ignored. In order to become peaceful with your scar and yourself you have to become familiar with this new part of your body.

You may hate it, hate what has happened to you and be extremely angry or sad. If you take this rage and focus it on your scar, you are only turning that intense emotion on a part of you that is already wounded, already hurt and trying to heal.

If you really cannot bear to touch your scar then either see a professional or do the massage through fabric or with a washcloth in the bath. However you do it does not matter so long as you touch the area and help the healing process.

This is not easy. This takes courage. To love is to accept, flaws and all. You would do it for those you treasure; please do it for yourself.

Massage Therapy

Chest draining massage

This massage helps move the lymph in the chest. If you have had full lymph removal on one side, give the other side extra attention. If both breasts and lymph nodes have been removed practice the deep breathing and "frog legs" lymph exercise more often.

> Use a little oil and firm, slow strokes. You do not need to use a lot of pressure here; the key is the regular movement which pushes the fluid in the chest towards the lymph nodes. To further activate the lymph it also helps to take full deep breaths.
>
> Starting at the base of the breastbone gently slide your fingers up between the breasts, over the chest area and over to one side, finishing in the armpit. Pause at the armpit and take a breath. Do this five times.
>
> After five full strokes pulse over the lymph nodes in the armpit, pressing gently with your fingers five times while breathing deeply.
>
> Now go under the breast again starting at the base of the breastbone and towards the armpit. Pause at the armpit for a deep belly breath and complete five full strokes.
>
> Finish the massage by gently rubbing along the sides of the breastbone where the ribs attach. Work between the ribs. These areas might be tender but ought to reduce once you get used to the massage.

Relieving breast congestion[10]

Congestion in the breast is most often experienced as painful soreness before your period, but it can also occur after surgery. The following massage is helpful for relieving breast congestion and note it does not involve massaging the breast itself.

> Identify the area of your breast that feels tender using a light touch with the pads of your fingers. When you find the most sensitive area maintain contact with your fingertips. Using your other hand, firmly massage the reflex area on your thigh. This is the area along the outside of the thigh from the knee to the hip. These are the lymphatic points that relate to the breast area.
>
> Using a circular motion, rub along the outer thigh just below your knee and work upwards to the hip. If an area on your thigh feels particularly tender, pay more attention to rubbing that spot. You might be shocked by how much it hurts! You will usually feel the soreness dissipate after a few seconds.
>
> When you get to the top of the leg stop and check your breast again for tenderness. If the pain is still there, repeat the rubbing from the knee up. Repeat the process each day until you feel the soreness has gone.

---

[10] Adapted from *Your Breasts: What every woman needs to know-now!* by Brian H. Butler

Professional massage

Certain situations require professional attention.

Lymphoedema:

After an operation there can be a sense of fullness under the arm which may be a fluid build-up on the chest wall. This is called a seroma, and the fluid may need to be drawn off by a nurse. In this situation lymphatic drainage massage is highly recommended to aid the working of the lymph system, and this requires a professional therapist. You can still help your lymph dramatically by following the 13 Lymph Activation exercises.

Cording:

This is a pain that feels like a tight rope running from the armpit down the arm to the wrist. It is thought to be caused by hardened lymph vessels or veins and can appear anywhere from six weeks to several months after surgery. Regular massage, stretching and physiotherapy help tremendously in the alleviation of cording.

My colleagues at London Bridge Hospital, Amanda Berlyn and Annette Dawson, are both skilled in scar massage techniques. Their contact details are in the Resources section. I will be providing advanced training for already qualified practitioners and as they complete the work I will list their details on the website www.LoveYourScar.com under Therapists.

Scar massage

Introduction

One of my visions is for scar massage to become a normal and regular part of post operative care so that the unnecessary pain and discomfort experienced by so many can be avoided. When I was receiving my massage training we were taught that touching the breast area on a woman crosses professional boundaries. In normal circumstances I fully respect this. However, this is simply not possible in the case of breast scar massage!

Several people tell me that they approached local therapists, but were unable to find any prepared to take them on, either because of where the scars were located or because they were a result of cancer surgery. Please send them to me for training. If there is a practitioner near you who will work on your scar I would encourage regular visits. Some patients visit me two to three times a month, while others come once every six weeks. It depends on how much work you are doing at home.

The fact remains that scars can be painful for years after surgery and require ongoing regular treatment. There are situations where you will want to see a professional; do what you can for yourself and ask for help if needed.

Self-administered massage – over to you

The physiology of scars has been explained and you understand the importance of freeing the fascia, so let's get to the techniques of scar massage.

It is important to note that scar release can be painful and the sensation is similar to burning or tingling as the fascia adhesions are pulled apart. If an area was previously numb and is now painful, this is excellent progress! Your body is waking up again.

You do not have to go beyond your pain threshold. Work gently, persistently and continue to make steady progress. You are not going to heal everything overnight so commit to the process long-term and congratulate yourself for sticking with it.

Massage your scars at least once a day ideally after your bath or shower when the skin is warm and pliable. Initially you may need more time for your massage as the affected area may be more extensive or painful. After a couple of weeks you will know where your sore spots are and where you need extra attention.

Making scar massage part of your daily routine is the best way to avoid adhesions and restrictions as well as keeping you in touch with your own healing process.

How soon should you begin scar massage?

While it is important not to work on an open wound or a scar that is too new, the sooner the area is gently stretched and massaged the better. Please, as a precaution, check with your breast care nurse or doctor before starting massage, especially if you have had complications such as infection or swelling. Working a scar too hard too soon may slow down healing.

Typically you should wait at least a month before massaging your scar with any significant pressure. Until then use a lighter touch simply to apply healing oils.

Other support measures include excellent nutrition, supplementation, homeopathy, deep breathing and regular stretching to keep the area pliable, mobile and assist the circulation around the wound.

Scar Massage

Understand your start point

When a scar is first healing it may feel itchy, sensitive or painful as the tissues reconnect, especially the nerves. Others find their scars and the surrounding area are completely numb. Feel around and see where the skin feels normal and where it seems different somehow.

Write a detailed description in your recovery journal. If the area around the scar is hard, how far does the hardness go? Is there any cording? How much range of motion is there? Move your arm in several directions to discover where the adhesions may be. Have they travelled downwards? Some people have sore ribs after a mastectomy while others with more extensive scarring find an entire side of their body is tight.

If both breasts have been removed, gently roll your neck around and see if there is restriction in the neck. Do you experience a pulling sensation between your shoulders? Move your body and see where you are today: this is your starting point.

Prepare your mind

Before you begin the massage take a couple of minutes to release any negative emotions or stress. The impact of positive thinking on patient recovery is a well-documented phenomenon, recognized by healthcare professionals worldwide. This book is about sending positive energy and healing to your scar. If this is new and unfamiliar territory to you, this technique helps you access the emotion we're looking for.

Thinking of a person you love dearly, hold them in your mind and reflect on how much you love them. Let the love you feel for them resonate in your body. You may feel warmth or lightness in your chest.

In your mind, send that loving feeling to the person you are thinking of. At the same time, feel that exact love and healing energy coursing through you, going to your scars or any part of you that feels painful or tired. Let your body relax and melt.

As you do your massage and lymph exercises, try your best to love that part of you that is healing. Of course you will have emotional ties to your illness, your wound and the resultant scar. You need to adjust your mindset to make these positive. This may take some practice.

If you hear your inner voice criticizing you, your scar or your circumstance, firmly (in your mind) say 'STOP!' and immediately replace the negative soundtrack with something positive such as 'I am healing and improving daily.' The inner critic has no positive purpose so you might as well tell it to go away.

Scar Massage

Getting started

Use a small amount of oil or lotion and with your fingertips apply gentle pressure directly to the scar and surrounding area, tracing small circles.

Note the feelings and sensations both on and around the scar. There may be hardness, numbness, tingling or burning to varying degrees. You may find that the ends of the scars or a point where a drain was placed are particularly sensitive. These sensations will change with continued massage.

In time, some areas will go back to normal, while others may stay numb or sensitive for longer. This is fine. If you have had repeated surgeries the scars may take a bit more time to change. Trust that with consistent attention they will continue to improve.

If you find the initial contact painful ease off slightly with your pressure, but keep your fingers on the painful spot. You can release muscular tension with your breath so use it whenever you need to. Breathe deeply, slowly and fully right down into your belly. After two or three breaths you ought to notice the pain has subsided.

Continue with the circular motions, working to your own limits, simply becoming comfortable touching your scar and familiar with the sensations around it. Stay at this level for the first two weeks, encouraging circulation and awareness.

Going deeper

After two weeks of daily massages using small circles it is time to move on to deeper strokes, as long as you feel ready to do so. With deeper massage you will tend to use less oil during the massage, as you need a certain amount of friction to access the deeper tissues. Warm the area using just a drop or two of oil and the circular motions.

To go deeper, work across the scar using your thumb or index finger in a zigzag pattern: this helps to stretch the scar tissue, increase flexibility and reduce adhesions. You may want to hold the skin around the scar taut so you can access the deeper layers. Go with your intuition and pay particular attention to any areas that are harder or more painful.

Work the entire chest area from the collarbone to the bottom of the ribcage and from the breastbone to under the armpit. If you have an implant you will want to massage that to keep it soft. Be careful when massaging any areas where there is mesh.

Massaging scars on the back is more difficult as they are harder to reach. Do as much as you can and ask a loved one or friend to help you with the areas you cannot access.

Scars on the buttocks or thighs will be easier to work if you raise your foot either on a chair or the side of the bath. This stretches out the scar so again you can move to the deeper tissues.

Undoubtedly there will be times when you are going along smoothly and hit a spot so painful that it takes your breath away. This is perfectly normal and will lessen over time. Back off the painful spot and deep breathe through the pain. Often you will know you are about to hit a sensitive area as it will feel more congested, either a bit swollen or as though your fingers cannot move smoothly and easily across the area. Don't avoid that area - spend more time on it, and make sure you note in your journal where it is so you can later reflect and enjoy knowing you released that pain and healed it.

When you feel able, perhaps in another week or so, add some pressure to the massage strokes and take it as far as you can, again noting your progress. You do not need to attack the painful areas and will find that the more you relax the more you release. Spend up to twenty minutes on your massage session and then stop for the day. Marathon sessions of massage are not advised and may impede the healing process simply because you are asking your body to do too much at one time.

Do not get to caught up in perfecting the technique; rather become acquainted with your scar and watch for signs of healing such as better sensation, increased range of motion, less pain, softness etc. The key is to give **constant daily attention** to keep the area mobile and the fascia pliable. When you have finished your massage apply a healing balm of organic oils to the area.

A note on emotional release – it is very common to have emotions come to the surface when doing this work. If you find yourself about to swallow back tears, inhale very deeply and slowly, then slowly exhale audibly. Keep doing this regardless of the emotion that is rising to be released. With each exhale sense that those locked emotions are leaving you; leaving you in peace, leaving you in love, leaving you to heal.

> *CASE STUDY: professional scar release*
>
> ## Eve's story
>
> *"I was first introduced to Adrianna Holman about 18 months after my mastectomy having had a lumpectomy just three weeks earlier. After the mastectomy I developed an infection which was treated by antibiotics, but left the whole area around and below the scar tissue very tender. My surgeon recommended that I try to do some massage of the area, but I had obviously not really found the right technique and was trying to avoid the very area I should have been massaging.*
>
> *It was at this low point when I was finding it uncomfortable to wear a bra for any length of time and still had a lot of numbness that I met Adrianna. We discussed the problems I was encountering and she advised scar massage to help the healing process and reduce tenderness. At first I had weekly massage sessions and was also shown how to continue the massage at home.*
>
> *I saw a slow but continued improvement (having left it so long after the operation before starting treatment I think it took longer to have an effect). Eventually we settled on one session a month, sometimes every 6 weeks or so, and I continued to massage at home in between.*
>
> *Now, nearly six years after the original operation I am virtually pain free. I have almost no numbness and hard tissue areas and most of the scar tissue has been dissipated. Without the help and encouragement of Adrianna I do not think I could have achieved so much.*

Natural beauty alternatives

What you put on your skin ends up in your blood and goes to every cell in your body. If you're not convinced consider nicotine and hormone patches. When you are healing you want to reduce your overall chemical load. I will focus on the things you put on your skin but also consider how many chemicals you use in your household cleaning. There are many 'green' products now that reduce your chemical exposure thereby helping you and the environment as well.

I suggest several products for your scars from various companies. If you like the products think about changing all your personal care items over to the natural lines. I mix and match but everything I use is chemical free, including makeup and fragrance.

Some companies offer samples so it is worth contacting them to try before you buy. Otherwise visit your local health store and take home samples of the available testers in your own little numbered pots or small bottles. Record what you are trying and how your skin feels. Do a patch test on your wrist before applying to your scar. Even though natural skin products are sourced from plants and flowers your skin may be sensitive to some ingredients.

Avoid Paraffin or mineral oil

> *Globally available and highlighting the need for scar care, this popular oil is backed by a fantastic marketing campaign. I was so excited when I first saw it on the shelf. I eagerly scanned the ingredient list and…my heart sank.*
>
> *The main ingredient is something you'd be better off avoiding.*
>
> *Paraffinum Liquidum or liquid paraffin, also known as mineral oil, is a by-product in the distillation of petroleum to produce gasoline and other petroleum based products from crude oil.*
>
> *According to the Environmental Working Group, which reviews the safety of cosmetic ingredients, numerous studies show tumor formation in animals exposed to paraffin.* [11]
>
> *CancerHelpUK warns that contact with petroleum products such as paraffin and mineral oil increase the risk of non melanoma skin cancer.* [12]
>
> *Look at your bottles at home and if paraffin is listed – chuck it out.*

---

[11] Environmental Working Group website: www.cosmeticsdatabase.com

[12] CancerHelpUK website: www.cancerhelp.org.uk/type/skin-cancer/about/skin-cancer-risks-and-causes

Natural Beauty Alternatives

My research on natural cosmetics and personal care started over twenty-five years ago when trying to heal my dreadful eczema. Natural products have come a long way since then and you can find everything you need these days from lipstick to nail varnish as well as holistic facials. My suggestions are not at all exhaustive; they are simply lines that I have used and like both on a personal and professional basis. I have included some less expensive ranges so everyone can benefit from natural skin care.

I recommend you use the most potent healing formula you can immediately after surgery to give a high concentration of nourishment to your scar in the initial healing stages, at least for the first three months.

For maintenance you may wish to continue using the more powerful formulas or move to a simpler and therefore less expensive option.

Please note that some of the purer products, particularly those that are oil based, need to be stored in a cool, dry place to help them last as they have no preservatives. If you are using them very sparingly keep them in the fridge.

One of my colleagues at London Bridge Hospital, Annette Dawson,[13] has been working as a complementary therapist since 1993 and is qualified in a range of therapies (including phenomenal Reflexology). Annette suggests several base oils to use for their positive effect on wound healing and scars.

---

[13] See Resources - People

Annette's Favorites

Use these as base oils and add desired essential oils.

> **Comfrey oil** helps promote healthy scar formation as well as assisting in the prevention of swelling and local edema.
>
> **Calendula oil** is established as an aid to wound healing and is often used on burns, scalds and sun damage making it perfect for sore skin.
>
> **Rosehip oil** assists the synthesis of collagen due to vitamin C content, oxygenates the skin and repairs damaged skin and scars including keloid scars.
>
> **Sunflower seed oil** helps repair damaged skin.
>
> **Sweet almond oil** is excellent on itchy, sore, hardened and sensitive tissue.

Clinical trials of various plant oils

- **Calendula** (Marigold) has been shown to have potent wound healing when used in clinical studies. On the eighth day of healing the wound had closed by 90% in those treated with Calendula versus 51% in those not treated.[14]

---

[14] Preethi KC, Kuttan R, 2009. Wound healing activity of flower extract of Calendula officinalis. *Journal of Basic and Clinical Physical and Pharmacology*, 20(1):73-9.

- **Hypericum** (St John's Wort) applied topically after Cesarean section helped minimize the formation and therefore the appearance of the scar, reduced pain and itching and facilitated wound healing.[15]

- **Comfrey** (Symphytum) has distinct healing effects.[16]

- **Rosehip seed oil** is one of the most nourishing oils and has anti-inflammatory and antioxidant properties.[17]

- **Frankincense oil** (Boswellic acids) made significant improvements on skin in regards to roughness, fine lines, photoaging (sun or radiation damage) as well as promoting an increase in elasticity.[18] Frankincense has also been shown to have anti-inflammatory properties in a number of different diseases.[19]

---

[15] Samadi S, Khadivzadeh T, Emami A, Moosavi NS, Tafaghodi M, Behnam HR, 2010. The effect of Hypericum perforatum on the wound healing and scar of caesarean. *Journal of Alternative and Complementary Medicine*, 16(1):113-7.

[16] Barna M, Kucera A, Hladicova M, Kucera M., 2007. [Wound healing effects of a Symphytum herb extract cream (Symphytum x uplandicum NYMAN:): results of a randomized, controlled double-blind study]. *Wiener Medizinische Wochenschrift*. 157(21-22):569-74.

[17] Chrubasik C, Roufogalis BD, Muller-Ladner U, Chrubasik S, 2008. A systematic review on the Rosa canina effect and efficacy profiles. *Phytotherapy Research*, 22(6):725-33.

[18] Calzavara-Pinton P, Zane C, Facchinetti E, Capezzera R, Pedretti A., 2010. Topical Boswellic acids for treatment of photoaged skin. *Dermatological Therapy*, 23: Suppl 1:S28-32.

[19] Ammon, HP, 2002. [Boswellic acids (components of frankincense) as the active principle in treatment of chronic inflammatory diseases). *Wiener Medizinische Wochenschrift*, 152(15-16):373-8.

- **German chamomile** has shown to significantly decrease weeping in the wound area.[20] A remarkable study comparing the wound healing of Chamomile to corticosteroids showed that animals treated with chamomile had significantly faster wound healing in comparison to those treated with corticosteroids. The scientists concluded that chamomile dramatically promotes wound healing.[21]

---

[20] Glowania HJ, Raulin C, Swoboda M., 1987. [Effect of **chamomile** on wound healing – a clinical double-blind study]. *Zeitschrift fur Hautkrankheiten*, 62(17):1262-1267-71.

[21] Martins, MD, Marques MM, Bussadori SK, Martins MA, Pavesi VC, Mesquita-Ferrari RA, Fernandes KP., 2009. Comparative analysis between **Chamomilla recutita** and corticosteroids on wound healing. An in vitro and in vivo study. *Phytotherapy Research,* 23(2):274-8.

Skin Deep Toxicity Rating of Natural Products

Before discussing the individual natural skin care lines I would like to draw attention to the Environmental Working Group[22] which rates the safety of cosmetics. I researched my favorite Dr.Hauschka products to see what rating they received. To my shock I noticed several scored as highly toxic. I investigated.

'Fragrance' or 'Parfum' is given a very high toxicity rating on the (American) website. Unfortunately and confusingly, EU law requires even 100% natural essential oils to be labeled as 'Fragrance'. The rating system for the website puts safe natural oils in the same category as synthetic chemical fragrance when clearly they are worlds apart. I found this misleading and unfair to the companies who have made an extraordinary effort to be non-toxic.[23]

It seems that the Environmental Working Group needs to rectify their rating system taking EU law into consideration if including European lines. You can find the Dr.Hauschka response to the rating system on Skin Deep here.[24] If you want to know what is in your products, contact the company directly and ask. You are the consumer and you have a right to know.

---

[22] www.cosmeticsdatabase.com

[23] Dr.Hauschka has invested over 45 years providing high quality, rigorously tested, natural and effective face and body care preparations which actually exceed Government legislation around the world.

[24] www.drhauschka.co.uk/skincare/brand/skin-deep

Inlight Organic Skin Care

I was curious about this range after reading the incredible ingredients listed in their Organic Line Softener. It had everything I could think of as regards healing herbs and flowers and then some. I decided to visit Cemon Homeopathics who make Inlight[25] organic skin care and took a trip to lovely Cornwall. I met with the team and the formulator Dr. Spiezia who is a medical doctor, homeopath and herbalist with thirty years of scientific research experience. His aim is to provide pure and healing skin care safe enough to eat. The company's philosophy is to respect and work in harmony with nature to achieve great beauty. They are environmentally aware and very sweetly donate their leftover herbs to the cows at Roskilly's organic farm, making for some happy and beautiful bovines.

Dr. Spiezia gave me a tour of the different organic flowers and herbs in the collection, passionately explaining the healing properties of each and how they are used in the products. Each Inlight product is hand-crafted through a combination of traditional methods and modern scientific expertise acquired through years of theoretical and empirical study by Dr. Spiezia. The raw materials are worked as little as possible in order to maintain their natural integrity and the oil-based extraction method concentrates key nutrients such as chlorophylls, fat soluble vitamins and anthocyanins (antioxidant flavonoids pigments) into the products.

---

[25] See Resources - Products

Natural Beauty Alternatives

The organic oils are poured over various herbs and flowers and left to infuse. The powerful herbal and floral properties synergize with the oil base and are pressed and filtered until a pure oil infusion remains. Every stage of the process is certified organic by the Soil Association and is completely cruelty free. Inlight has received several awards (the Organic Line Softener was Highly Commended in the Natural Health Beauty Awards 2009) and I have used several of the products personally. I've been using the Organic Line Softener with excellent results during scar massage.

Lisa, a patient, reviews the product:

"Following my mastectomy and reconstructive surgery I was very interested in finding a product that would help to reduce the size and appearance of my two scars. I have been using Inlight Organic Line Softener for over six weeks now and am very pleased with the results. My scars do seem to be reducing and they feel really smooth."

The Inlight Organic Line Softener contains so many nourishing ingredients in the base alone: **Shea butter** and **macadamia oil** provide Vitamins A and E plus essential fatty acids; **carrot oil** rich in beta-carotene assists skin restoration; **evening primrose oil** and **sunflower oil** have regenerative properties; **jojoba oil** promotes skin elasticity vital to scar treatment and **olive oil** soothes the skin.

On top of the highly recuperative base are the carefully chosen added plant extracts: **Gota kola, marigold** and **plantain** all promote skin healing by stimulating cellular regeneration, **bilberry** is an antioxidant, **lemon** and **rose** are astringent, **horsetail** and **nettle** help the skin restore mineral balance and **lavender, patchouli** and **rose geranium** are known for their anti-inflammatory properties. The 100% organic and GM free ingredients in this balm nourish, regenerate and restore the skin while protecting it from inflammation.

One of my patients had a terrible reaction to the petroleum based scar oil mentioned earlier and I suggested she try the Inlight Organic Line Softener. Once she switched her skin rash completely cleared from the chest area within days and she noticed her scar became much softer and smoother. All the ladies giggle when I ask how they are finding the cream saying it helps so much, smells so gorgeous and that they dot a little bit around their eyes as well for good measure.

Karen also reviews the product:

"I have had two hip re-surfacing operations this year which left me with two 19cm scars. The first scar was closed with dissolvable stitching and I used Bio-oil regularly to help the healing process. After about three months there were no noticeable changes to the color or texture of the scar. It was then suggested by a friend that I try Inlight Organic Line Softener. I started to use this sparingly nearly every day and within just a few weeks the redness had all but disappeared and the skin texture was smoother.

My second operation was closed with clips and on this occasion the operated area was very sore and numb. I used the Organic Line Softener straight away on this scar and within a few weeks the skin became soft, less numb to the touch and the red line started to diminish. It is now nearly twelve weeks since my second operation and I am still using the Line Softener regularly, the redness is certainly diminishing, the skin is lovely and soft and the muscle underneath the skin seems a lot less hard and lumpy."

Inlight Offer and Charitable Donation

Inlight has generously offered to give a **30% discount on their Organic Line Softener** through a cut-out voucher at the back of *Love Your Scar*. Send it to the company with a cheque or phone with card details.

With the voucher the Organic Line Softener will cost £35.42 instead of the regular retail price of £50.60 (at the time of publication).

Inlight Organic Line Softener will be available from the online store at a 20% discount during Breast Cancer Awareness month (October 2010).

For every Organic Line Softener sold during October 2010 Inlight will donate £1 to the charity **Yes to Life** - www.yestolife.org.uk

Furthermore they will donate 10p to Yes to Life on an ongoing basis with each purchase of the Organic Line Softener.

I am so touched by their desire to help women with scars feel better faster and also of their support of Yes to Life. I hope you will try the Inlight Organic Line Softener on your scar as it really is an exceptional formula.

Inlight has a complete range of 100% sumptuous skin care for face and body.

Dr.Hauschka

Dr.Hauschka Skin Care[26] (under the WALA umbrella) boasts over 130 natural beauty products as well as a Dr.Hauschka Med range created for specific needs. Many of the medicinal herbs used in Dr.Hauschka products are grown in WALA's own gardens. Where possible the plants are grown biodynamically, organically or harvested in the wild.

I have to say I adore this range. From head to toe there is a Dr.Hauschka product made to beautify you. I use the gorgeous cosmetics as well as the face and body care products.

I was introduced to the power of Dr.Hauschka when searching for holistic facials in 2002. I visited Amanda Berlyn[27], a Dr. Hauschka aesthetician and winner of the 2005 British Beauty Awards. She explained that one of the fundamental principles behind Dr.Hauschka treatments is the activation of the lymph. The products and rhythmic application methods encourage lymph movement which naturally makes the skin dynamic, boosting circulation and activity.

Amanda is a member of the complementary therapy team at London Bridge Hospital and is experienced in scar massage as well as giving absolutely divine facials and body treatments using all Dr.Hauschka products.

---

[26] See Resources – Products

[27] See Resources - People

Natural Beauty Alternatives

Amanda's recommended Dr.Hauschka products

Rejuvenating Mask: This is excellent for skin cell renewal, improving the appearance of the scars as well as softening hardened skin tissue. It is not oily and absorbs easily. The highly nurturing plant oils and extracts infuse skin with moisture and antioxidants while calming sensitivities and redness. Use a small amount twice daily on the scar after massage.

Moor Lavender oil: This is a mix of olive oil and shea butter making it perfect for scar massage. Shea butter is naturally rich in Vitamin A and the moisturizing property is the same as that produced by the sebaceous glands in the skin. Lavender essential oil and moor (peat moss) extract provide comfort, protection and a sense of well-being to the sensitive or restless person. This would be of particular benefit to use for an evening massage if you are anxious or having trouble sleeping as the Lavender helps you relax.

Rhythmic Night Conditioner ampoules: These encourage proper hydration and revitalize pale, lifeless skin. This preparation supports the skin's natural 28-day process of renewal, restoring harmony during periods of imbalance or transition, such as times of stress. The Night Conditioner has the same sort of consistency as water and would be gently pressed into the scar. Definitely use at night for 28 days as soon as the scar has healed over and stopped weeping.

Neal's Yard Remedies

Neal's Yard Remedies (NYR)[28] has a strict 'NO' policy: no animal testing, no GMO ingredients, no parabens, no nano particles, no synthetic fragrances or colors, no silicones, no mineral oils, no phthalates, no EDTA, no propylene glycol (petroleum derivative), no carbomer (petroleum derivative) and no DEA.

NYR offer a completely bland lotion and ointment base so you can create your own specialized scar blend.

I contacted Susan Curtis, Medicines Director for Neal's Yard Remedies, for a recommendation on NYR products for scars.

Susan's Suggestions

- Calendula Macerated Oil
- Calendula Cream
- Hypericum and Calendula cream
- Comfrey Macerated Oil
- Rosehip seed oil
- Frankincense (Olibanum) essential oil: (dilute at 1-2% in a base oil such as calendula oil).
- Lavender essential oil: dilute as above

NYR will give you samples to take home and try.

---

[28] See Resources – Products

Trilogy

Trilogy[29] commissioned a clinical study to test the effect of Trilogy Certified Organic Rosehip Oil (TORO) on scars. The study was conducted at an independent laboratory in Australia during 2009, in accordance with ICH Guidelines for Good Clinical Practice.

Ten test subjects between the ages of 20 and 60 had scars in different stages of healing ranging from very new to well-established and from mild to severe intensity. No other skincare products were permitted in the skin area during the study and no adverse reactions were observed. TORO was applied twice a day and assessments taken at four, eight and twelve weeks.

All ten test subjects reported an improvement in the overall appearance of their scars as well as improvements in softness and evenness of scars after twelve weeks of use. Changes in the scar were all assessed by an expert and the results show a 41% improvement in the color of scars, a 27% improvement in the appearance of scars and a 26% improvement in the visible area of the scars.

Rosehip oil is naturally rich in Beta-carotene and Lycopene, both powerful antioxidants that assist in cell renewal and repair and protect against stress as well as Omega-3 and Omega-6 Essential Fatty Acids (EFAs) which improve skin softness and elasticity.

---

[29] See Resources – Products

Weleda

As well as using organic natural skin care products on your scar I would really like to see you use them all over. These next two are purse friendly as well as kind on your skin.

A lovely and extensive range, (and another one of my personal favorites), Weleda[30] was founded over eighty years ago by Dr. Rudolph Steiner and holds to the philosophy "when we say all natural we mean all natural." Weleda came about when farmers in the early 20th century noticed a decline in the health of their crops and livestock. Steiner, renowned philosopher and natural scientist, created the principles that now define Biodynamic agriculture and the Weleda philosophy.

He described a farm as a complete organism in its own right. Farmers used composting and natural fertilization and pest control rather than relying on chemicals or growth hormones. The natural rhythms of the sun, moon and planets guided the farmers for the optimal time for planting, crop rotation and harvesting. Biodynamic agriculture involves growing to organic standards, nurturing the soil and respecting the natural rhythms and vitality of the plants. The plants are picked at the peak of potency to enhance healing and restore radiance.

---

[30] See Resources – Products

Skin Blossom

The Organic Bloom range by Skin Blossom[31] has been specially created to contain organic and skin-friendly ingredients at an affordable price. The range is certified by the Soil Association for organic purity as well as the Vegan Society meaning it contains no animal ingredients or testing. Each product has been carefully formulated using plant extracts and oils to deliver key nutrients and protection to skin. Organic Bloom products are suitable for all skin types, even the most sensitive skin.

Nelsons Scar Cream

Nelsons Scar Cream[32] is a bit different in that it contains a homeopathic remedy as well as nourishing oils. This formula is a gentle blend of Rosehip oil, Vitamin E oil, Calendula tincture and Thiosiniminum 6x (homeopathic remedy for helping scars) in a paraben/paraffin free base cream. Using this cream topically as well as taking homeopathic remedies internally seems to help speed along healing with my patients who have tried it.

---

[31] See Resources – Products
[32] See Resources – Products

Be a curious shopper and make sure whatever you put on your skin is natural, nourishing and contains as few chemicals as possible if any at all. This includes shampoo, makeup, nail varnish, deodorant, toothpaste and all other personal care items you use regularly. Be a little obsessive with your beauty... your health is worth it.

Recommended Reading:

- *The Green Beauty Bible* by Sarah Stacey and Josephine Fairley (2009, London: Kyle Cathie Publishing)

- *Look Great Naturally... without ditching the lipstick* by Janey Lee Grace (2010, London: Hay House UK)

Nutrition

We've never had it so good?

The World Health Organization puts poor diet is at the top of its list of cancer causes, second only to smoking. Half of all cancers are down to poor food choices.[33] When I started researching breast cancer and nutrition I found consistently contradictory medical research. Pro soy, anti soy, pro dairy, anti dairy, pro fat but only the right kind, pro fruit but anti sugar... This medical quote sums it up: "Dietary contribution to breast cancer risk, recurrence, and progression remains incompletely understood." [34]

I feel we are bombarded by potentially too much information about what we should eat and what we should avoid. I don't know about you but I find it terribly confusing when each expert provides clinical evidence stating why their diet is the direct route to health and yet it conflicts with what last month's expert said.

The problem is that we do not all fit into the same box and this includes our dietary needs. Given this I appeal to you to use your common sense.

---

[33] World Health Organization website
http://www.who.int/dietphysicalactivity/publications/facts/cancer/en

[34] Dave B, Wynne R, Su Y, Korourian S, Chang JC, Simmen RC., 2010. Enhanced mammary progesterone receptor-a isoform activity in the promotion of mammary tumor progression by dietary soy in rats. *Nutrition and Cancer*, 62(6):774-82.

Everyone is different. This means you have to pay attention to how your body feels.

Food gives you energy. If you feel sleepy, bloated, foggy or cranky after a meal that is a clear indication something you ate did not agree with you. If you really want to know what works for you, keep a food diary and write down everything you eat and drink and describe how you feel emotionally and physically in detail for at least ten days. If you discover you feel bloated after eating toast, eliminate it for a couple of weeks. If you have an energy crash after eating fruit on its own try having it with nuts. Experiment and find out what works best for you as an individual.

Diets used to be much simpler, based on ingredients you could pronounce and usually involved something that grew from the ground, ran on the ground, swam or flew. In the past couple of generations there has been an explosion in food processing. Our taste buds have been manipulated by the food industry to crave fat, sugar and salt.[35] Our foods contain cocktails of chemicals - artificial coloring and flavoring, preservatives, multiple pesticides - and our brains are overloaded with skilful marketing encouraging us to choose these so called foods.

I am not going to suggest that a carrot stick will satisfy a chocolate craving and it is ridiculous to even try that approach. However we have to get back to the healthy foods as a base and if you tend to eat a lot of junk it will take some effort initially. Once you are actually getting nourishment from your food then you can enjoy nutrient rich chocolate

---

[35] Kessler, David, 2009. *The end of overeating*, London, England: Penguin Group.

(yes it exists) when those cravings hit. Chances are once you eat a healthier diet you won't crave it quite so much. It's all about the balance.

One area that is really non-negotiable when healing from surgery is junk food. Be ruthless and cut it out completely. The main harmful foods are overly refined flours, sugar and trans-fats. An Italian review of cancer cases dating back to the 1990s indicates that following a Mediterranean diet can help minimize cancer risk. The findings show that using olive oil in place of saturated fat is protective and eating whole grains reduces the risk of various cancers whereas refined grains and high sugar diets increase risk of cancer. Fish is protective while frequent intake of red meat is directly related to the growth of abnormal masses of tissue.[36]

The traditional Okinawan diet (in Southern Japan) is vegetable and fruit heavy (therefore phytonutrient and antioxidant rich) and has minimal amounts of meat, refined grains, saturated fat, sugar, salt and full-fat dairy products. This type of diet is likely to reduce the risk of some cancers and other chronic diseases. The Okinawan diet is low in fat intake, particularly in terms of saturated fat, and high in antioxidant-rich yet low calorie orange-yellow root vegetables such as sweet potatoes as well as plenty of green leafy vegetables. Why mention the Okinawan diet? These people have a long average life expectancy, high numbers of centenarians, and a low risk of age-associated diseases.[37]

---

[36] Bosetti C, Pelucchi C LaVecchia C, 2009. Diet and cancer in Mediterranean countries: carbohydrates and fats. *Public Health Nutrition*, 12(9A):1595-600.

[37] Willcox DC, Willcox BJ, Todoriki H, Suzuki M., 2009. The Okinawan diet: health implications of a low-calorie, nutrient-dense, antioxidant-rich dietary pattern low in glycemic load. *Journal of the American College of Nutrition*, 28 Suppl:500S-516S.

Highly processed foods such as crisps, rice cakes, biscuits and white bread do not give us enough nutrition, so the body is not satisfied and we feel compelled to eat more, consuming not only an excess of calories, but also more of the very foods that cause many health problems.

Many if not most people eating standard western diets suffer from blood sugar imbalances due to the highly processed, quick release foods widely available. Sugar gives us a fast 'high' followed by an almighty crash sending us wildly in search of a quick high again. Besides the extraordinary amount of sugar and salt now common in our food we need to look at one of the most dangerous products in our food. Out of all the information I present on diet and nutrition, if you only take one tiny bit to heart it is this...

AVOID Trans fats!

Trans fatty acids (TFAs) are chemically altered oils, are not essential fats and definitely do not promote good health. A seven year study published in the *American Journal of Epidemiology* found that a high level of TFAs is probably one **major factor** contributing to an increased risk of invasive breast cancer in women.[38]

The UK Faculty of Public Health and The Royal Society for Public Health have now called to eliminate TFAs by 2011, as cited in *The British Medical Journal*. They state that it has been proven that industrially-produced TFAs can damage health and that **there is no safe level of consumption.**[39]

TFAs and hydrogenated fats have commercial advantages as they increase the shelf life of food and don't cost much to produce. The main sources of TFAs are deep fried foods, fast foods, packaged snacks (Ramen noodles and soup cups, microwave popcorn), margarine, shortening and baked goods (cakes, cookies, biscuits, donuts), frozen pies, pot pies, waffles and pizzas to name a few.

---

[38] Chajes V, Thiebaut ACM, Rotival M, Gauthier E, Maillard V, Boutron-Ruault M-C, Joulin V, Lenoir GM, Clavel-Chapelon F, 2008. Association between Serum *trans*-Monounsaturated Fatty Acids and Breast Cancer Risk in the E3N-EPIC Study. *American Journal of Epidemiology*, 167(11):1312-1320.

[39] Dariush Mozaffarian D, Stampfer MJ, 2010. Removing industrial *trans* fats from foods. *British Medical Journal*, 340:c1826.

Many large corporations are phasing TFAs out of their foods but some are dragging their heels. If a product is super cheap you'd better take a look at the ingredients. There is most likely a shortcut on nutrition somewhere.

Read labels carefully.

It is usually written on the packet if a product does not contain trans fats or hydrogenated fats. If your favorite biscuit still uses cheap altered fats, write to the company and urge them to use safer fats. Don't underestimate the power of the consumer. If enough people make noise, the companies will change.

TFAs dramatically increase bad cholesterol levels (while decreasing good cholesterol levels), increase systemic inflammation, cell dysfunction, irregular heartbeat, insulin resistance, diabetes development, cardiovascular risk and abdominal fat which is considered more dangerous to health....

Yikes!

Organic Food

I am a vocal advocate for organic food, especially, absolutely when in suboptimal health or recovery. Human epidemiological studies and experimental animal data strongly suggest that organochloride pesticides have a positive correlation to breast cancer risk.[40] DDT has been found to be undisputedly associated with breast cancer risk.[41] One horrific study showed that women exposed to DDT as small children developed breast cancer decades later.[42] Do we really know what the multiple combinations of different agricultural chemicals are doing to us?

In a best case scenario **all** your food would be organically sourced. Reviews of multiple studies show that organic varieties **do** provide significantly greater levels nutrients than non-organic varieties of the same foods, particularly vitamin C, iron, magnesium and phosphorus. Organics are also significantly lower in nitrates and pesticide residues. In addition, with the exception of wheat, oats, and wine, organic foods typically provide greater levels of a number of important antioxidant

---

[40] Fénichel P, Brucker-Davis F, 2008. Environmental endocrine disrupters and breast cancer: new risk factors? [Article in French] *Gynécologie, Obstétrique & Fertilité*, 36(10) :969-77.

[41] Shakeel MK, George PS, Jose J, Jose J, Mathew A, 2010. Pesticides and breast cancer risk: a comparison between developed and developing countries. *Asian Pacific Journal of Cancer Prevention*, 11(1):173-80.

[42] Cohn BA, Wolff MS, Cirillo PM, Sholtz RI., 2007. DDT and breast cancer in young women: new data on the significance of age at exposure. *Environmental Health Prospectives*, 115(10):1406-14.

phytochemicals (anthocyanins, flavonoids, and carotenoids).[43] A ten-year study on organically grown vs. conventionally grown tomatoes showed that organically grown tomatoes had levels of quercetin and kaempferol (both flavonoids essential to rebuilding good health) respectively 79% and 97% higher than the conventionally grown. Even better, the levels of flavonoids increased over time in organic samples whereas conventional samples did not significantly vary. The nutrient increase corresponded with increasing amounts of organic matter naturally accumulating in the soil. Manure application was reduced once soils in the organic systems reached equilibrium levels of organic matter. The organic soil needed less treatment yet the tomatoes had more nutrients.[44] The Soil Association[45] gives five more excellent reasons to go organic:

1. Your well-being

Organic food standards ban hydrogenated fats and controversial additives including aspartame (artificial sweetener), tartrazine (food coloring E102 or FD&C Yellow #5) and MSG (monosodium glutamate is a flavor enhancer). No need to worry about any of that in your food.

2. The environment

Organic farming releases less greenhouse gases than non-organic farming. Choosing to buy organic, local and seasonal food can

---

[43] Crinnion, WJ, 2010. Organic foods contain higher levels of nutrients, lower levels of pesticides, and may provide health benefits for the consumer. *Alternative Medicine Review*, 15(1):4-12.

[44] Mitchell AE, Hong YJ, Koh E, Barrett DM, Bryant DE, Denison RF, Kaffka S., 2007. Ten-year comparison of the influence of organic and conventional crop management practices on the content of flavonoids in tomatoes. *Journal of Agricultural and Food Chemistry*, 55(15):6154-9

[45] Soil Association website - www.soilassociation.org

significantly reduce your carbon footprint. This counts in a far reaching way, supporting local farmers, reducing pollution for future generations and making a stand against unnecessary harm to the planet.

3. Animal welfare

Organic standards insist that animals are given plenty of space and fresh air guaranteeing a truly free-range life. All aspects of animal welfare are tightly controlled for the duration of the animal's life. Emphasis is on keeping the animal healthy rather than using drugs to treat disease. Organic farmers provide appropriate nutritious feed, ensure easy access to the outdoors and keep stress to a minimum for the animals.

Organic animals cannot be given growth promoting hormones, regular doses of antibiotics or genetically modified (GM) feed. If an animal becomes sick it is treated using homeopathic and complementary remedies unless a vet says antibiotics are needed. If an animal is treated with antibiotics a set period of time has to pass before products from that animal can be sold as organic. This time period is on average *three times as long* as those required by law for non-organic food.

4. Protecting wildlife

Organic farms are havens for wildlife which we desperately need as over the past fifty years the UK has seen a drastic decline in wildlife. Organic farming depends on a diverse ecosystem to maintain soil fertility and keep pests naturally under control. Organic farms provide homes for bees, birds, bats and butterflies all of whom play a vital role in the planet's survival. The UK Government's own advisors found that plant, insect and bird life is up to 50% greater on organic farms. As no chemicals are used (non-organic farming uses around 31,000 tons of chemicals annually in the UK alone) organic farming preserves life.

5. GM-free

Genetically modified crops and ingredients are banned under organic standards. A 2008 poll from Friends of the Earth showed that 87% of the UK public does not want GM foods in the supermarkets. Currently no GM crops are grown in the EU for human consumption but GM animal feed provides a back-door entry for GM products into the EU. Even worse is that the current rules say meat and dairy products from animals fed on GM animal feed do not need to be labeled as GM.[46]

Organic farming is about producing food that is good for you, good for animals and good for the environment. It is a total system of production that works in harmony with nature rather than fighting it with chemicals, fertilizers and antibiotics. Organic is a more sustainable choice, especially as around 30% of the average consumer's carbon footprint comes from food choices.

Probably the biggest complaint against organic food is that it is too expensive. But compared to what - poor health? Once enough people choose organic food the cost will drop. You must remember that each time you shop, you vote. Big business is going to sway to consumer demand or else go out of business. You have great power in your purse. One organic delivery company, Riverford, regularly compares their organic vegetable box prices against online prices for the equivalent organic produce from Tesco, Sainsbury's and Waitrose. They have

---

[46] Friends of the Earth website -   www.foe.co.uk

Nutrition

consistently come out cheaper, normally by about 20% (and they have free delivery). In March 2010 their 'roots + greens vegbox' was 44% cheaper than in supermarkets and the 'large vegbox' was 43% cheaper.[47] I also like this company's attitude towards the environment.

On average 80% of their fruits and vegetables are grown in the UK which is much higher than for any supermarket and most box schemes and supports local farms. Riverford never airfreights as air freight causes 40 to 50 times the CO_2 emissions of sea freight. Imports for Riverford come primarily from France, Spain and Morocco to cover the demands for year-round tomatoes, apples and peppers as well as citrus and bananas. Growing tomatoes out of season using hothouses in the UK can be more than ten times as damaging to the environment as trucking them in from Southern Europe.[48]

Remind yourself why you are buying organic: health, humane treatment of animals and environmental protection. Choosing organic avoids polluting your body with pesticides, additives, antibiotic residuals and GM products. Organically reared animals have had the highest standards of welfare with no factory farming, growth hormones and needless drugs. Choosing to buy organic food means you have supported a system of agriculture that uses natural resources sustainably, has less of a negative impact on the environment and encourages wildlife and biodiversity.

---

[47] Riverford Organic Veg website - www.riverford.co.uk
[48] Riverford Organic Veg website - www.riverfordenvironment.co.uk

Go organic as much as you can especially for fragile foods (lettuce and strawberries), meat and dairy. At the very least buy these twelve foods organically as they tend carry to highest amount of residual pesticides:

- apples and pears
- nectarines, cherries and peaches
- strawberries
- grapes
- carrots and celery
- lettuce and kale
- bell peppers

I highly recommend you see the movie Food Inc., directed by Robert Kenner, for a more in-depth look at conventional farming vs. locally grown organic farming to see the true cost of cheap food.

Also be sure to look in the Resources section under 'Food' for three organic delivery companies here in the UK. If you cannot find organic foods easily near you, go for seasonal fresh, ideally locally grown foods. Visit farmers markets and talk to the farmers about their pesticide use. Explore and investigate your options. You have choices.

Eat more fresh food

As a first step add **in one portion of fresh fruit per day and two portions of vegetables per day**, (on top of what you already eat) building up to at least seven portions of fruit and vegetables per day, every day. Seven? Yes, at least seven. Ten is better still. This is not as difficult as it sounds and the super smoothie recipe takes care of several of those portions in one swoop. Every time you eat, whether making a full meal or just a snack, make sure one or two items are fresh. It's that easy. Remember you are building a new you after surgery and optimal nutrition is what you want to build your foundation on.

You will find your taste buds start craving fresher foods and will enjoy the lightness and energy in your body rather than gas, heartburn and sluggish bowels. As you make the changes over to more fruits and vegetables you may feel hungrier. I would advise initially to drink a glass of water and wait five minutes. If you are truly hungry, eat! Just make a clever choice and reach for the healthier option more often than not and simply by default your body and moods will improve.

Reducing or eliminating junk foods of sugar, refined flour and unhealthy fats may feel like punishment but really it isn't. You aren't losing your "treats"; you are just finding new ones to support your healing. When you first stop eating junk you can feel a bit sick as your body cleans house. The first couple of days are the worst so plan to take extra rest and drink plenty of water.

Load up with Vitamin C

We all know fruits and vegetables are good for us but maybe we aren't so sure why that is. These foods are critical to healing as their nutrients strengthen blood vessels and connective tissues as well as boost the immune system. Fruits and vegetables are high in vitamin C (ascorbic acid) amongst other nutrients. Brazilian scientists found ascorbic acid **acted positively on every stage of the healing process** –

- Assisting the immune system
- Increasing the tissue and new blood vessels critical for wound healing
- Stimulating the synthesis of thicker and more organized collagen fibers in the wounds.

Vitamin C has anti-inflammatory and healing effects which guaranteed a suitable environment for faster skin repair.[49]

Eat more foods rich in this essential nutrient. The next page has a chart of foods high in Vitamin C.

---

[49] Lima CC, Pereira AP, Silva JR, Oliveira LS, Resck MC, Grechi CO, Bernardes MT, Olímpio FM, Santos AM, Incerpi EK, Garcia JA., 2009. Ascorbic acid for the healing of skin wounds in rats. *Brazilian Journal of Biology*, 69(4):1195-201.

Foods High in Vitamin C

FRUIT	VEGETABLE
- citrus	- bell peppers
- rosehips	- spring greens
- strawberries	- artichokes
- blackcurrants	- spinach
- guava	- red cabbage
- lychees	- parsley
- goji berries	- kale
- kiwi	- broccoli
- papaya	- Brussels sprouts
- peach	- cauliflower
- mango	- mange tout peas
	- potatoes have vitamin C (But not as much as kale. Eat your kale).

Super Greens

Leading the pack of all healthy foods are the dark leafy greens furthermore referred to as greens.

Greens are full of nutrients, particularly a group of B vitamins called folates which maintain DNA stability. Worryingly there is a widespread deficiency of folate in humans and this deficiency has been implicated in the development of several cancers including cancer of the colon, ovary, breast, pancreas, cervix, brain and lung. Data from the majority of human studies suggests that people who habitually eat foods high in folate, (i.e. greens) have a significantly reduced risk of developing colon polyps or cancer.[50]

Super Greens include kale, broccoli, romaine lettuce, red and green leaf lettuce, spinach, endive, chard, celery, bok choy, asparagus, arugula, carrot tops, collard greens, escarole, frisee, mizuna, mustard greens and radicchio.

---

[50] Duthie SJ, 2010. Folate and cancer: how DNA damage, repair and methylation impact on colon carcinogenesis. *Journal of Inherited Metabolic Disease*, June 11 [Epub ahead of print]

Antioxidants

Fruits and vegetables are also high in antioxidant substances called **phytonutrients**. Scientists found that antioxidant plant extracts, including green and black tea, carotenoids and many flavonoids in fruit and vegetables can protect skin from irradiation induced cancer.[51]

I would like to highlight one antioxidant in particular – CoEnzymeQ10 or CoQ10. This nutrient benefits everyone, especially those recovering from surgery.

One study reported that a deficiency in CoQ10 resulted in oxidative stress and cell damage, exactly what you **do not want** when healing from cancer.[52] Furthermore in animal studies CoQ10 was found to increase endurance and stave off fatigue which again would be highly supportive of the healing process.[53]

The next page gives a table outlining some key antioxidants.

---

[51] Reuter J, Merfort I, Schempp CM, 2010. Botanicals in dermatology: an evidence-based review. *American Journal of Clinical Dermatology*, 11(4):247-67.

[52] Quinzii CM, López LC, Gilkerson RW, Dorado B, Coku J, Naini AB, Lagier-Tourenne C, Schuelke M, Salviati L, Carrozzo R, Santorelli F, Rahman S, Tazir M, Koenig M, Dimauro S, Hirano M, 2010. Reactive oxygen species, oxidative stress, and cell death correlate with level of CoQ10 deficiency. *The FASEB Journal: official publication of the Federation of American Societies for Experimental Biology*, [Epub ahead of print]

[53] Fu X, Ji R, Dam J, 2010. Anti fatigue effect of coenzyme Q10 in mice. *Journal of Medicinal Food*, 13(1):211-5.

Star-performer Antioxidants

Antioxidant	*What it does*	*Found in these foods*
Quercetin	Anti-inflammatory action which supports post-operative recovery.	Apples, red onions, green tea, broccoli, leafy greens, tomatoes and berries
Carotenoids (converted by the body into Vitamin A)	Essential for wound healing and proper immune functioning.	Food sources high in carotenoids are usually red, orange or yellow- carrots, apricots, winter squash, mangos, plums, tomatoes, pumpkin and sweet potatoes.[54]
Selenium	Selenium-enriched plants have been identified as having anti-cancer properties.[55]	Garlic and onions Broccoli and wild leek
Curcumin	Anti-inflammatory, antioxidant and anti-cancer properties.[56]	Curcumin is the active ingredient of the spice turmeric. It has been used in Indian and African medicine for centuries.
Coenzyme Q10 (CoQ10)	An antioxidant with a fundamental role in cellular energy with numerous known health benefits.	Meat, fish and nuts (contain high levels) Dairy, vegetables, fruit and cereals (lower levels)

---

[54] The body absorbs carotenoids better when eaten or cooked with a little oil.

[55] Arnault I & Auger J., 2006. Seleno-compounds in garlic and onion. *Journal of Chromatography* 1112(1-2):23-30.

[56] Epstein J, Sanderson IR, Macdonald TT, 2010. Curcumin as a therapeutic agent: the evidence from in vitro, animal and human studies. *The British Journal of Nutrition*, 103(11):1545-57.

Omega 3 foods

Although some fats are bad for us, others are extremely good for us. Our bodies need good fats known as **essential fatty acids**, especially Omega 3 fats. These are quite literally essential to good health and wound healing, particularly right after surgery as they have anti-inflammatory properties and increase collagen.[57]

Foods high in Omega 3 fats
Oily fish such as salmon, sardines and mackerel
Dark leafy greens
Soya beans
Walnuts
Flax seeds, hempseed and pumpkin seeds

There has been much debate over fish vs. plants as the ideal source of Omega 3. To cover both sides you can eat fatty fish like salmon, mackerel and sardines and add a daily dose of flaxseed to your diet, either ground freshly every day or soaked in water overnight. While healing take an Omega 3 supplement to ensure you are receiving enough of this vital nutrient in case your diet falls short.

---

[57] One clinical study reports that Omega 3 fatty acids have a non-invasive, therapeutic potential to affect cutaneous wound healing and another study states that Omega 3 fatty acids increased collagen synthesis and the overall percentage of collagen produced in wounds.

General food groups

Grains

Eat whole grains such as brown rice, whole oats, millet and whole grain breads. Whole grain breads are denser and retain the fiber which is important for the gastrointestinal tract. Remember fiber also slows down the release of the carbohydrate in the grain. Try different grains such as amaranth and quinoa.

Some people are sensitive to gluten. If you feel bloated or sleepy after eating wheat, rye, barley or oats stop them for two weeks and see if symptoms improve. Eat them sparingly *if at all* if you do have a problem.

Meat

The China Study[58] comes to the conclusion that the best diet for overall health is a whole food, plant-based one. The authors suggest any meat or dairy to be detrimental to health. Indeed the incidence of some cancers may be lower in fish eaters and vegetarians than in meat eaters.

A study on diet and cancer followed 61,566 British men and women, comprising of 32,403 meat eaters, 8562 fish eaters (but no meat) and 20,601 vegetarians. In a twelve year follow up there were 3350 incident cancers of which 2204 were among meat eaters, 317 among fish eaters and 829 among vegetarians.[59] Figuring the math, out of the total amount

---

[58] Campbell T. Colin & Campbell II, T.M., 2006. *The China Study*. Dallas:BenBella Books

[59] Key TJ, Appleby PN, Spencer EA, Travis RC, Allen NE, Thorogood M, Mann JI, 2009. Cancer incidence in British vegetarians. *British Journal of Cancer,* 101(1):192-7.

Nutrition

of cancer cases 65% were meat eaters. There was no mention of lifestyle, smoking, drinking, family history etc. which is why I hesitate to make a blanket statement about eating meat. Of all the research I have read on meat and cancer the general conclusion is that a high intake of red meat contributes to an increased risk of cancer. No one seems to state what a high intake is so I do not know if it is three times a day or three times a week. As there is no scientific conclusion my suggestion is that if you eat meat, find the freshest cut you can, ideally sourced locally and as I've mentioned before, organic or at the very least, free-range. Simply eat less of it, avoid processed meats (salami, bologna) and choose leaner cuts or opt for more poultry and game over beef and lamb.

I know organic meat costs more, sometimes a lot more. The idea is to use it sparingly, more as a seasoning rather than a huge slab of meat on your plate with a smattering of vegetables. Make the vegetables the largest part of the meal with meat used more for flavor than substance. That way a high quality, highly flavorful portion of meat will go much further.

If you don't like meat or you want to completely cut it out of your diet please make sure you get adequate protein as this is necessary for healing. Use fish, pulses, soy foods and protein powders. Mix up your diet and get a variety of different types of protein sources. I would not rely too heavily on any one source. Even though they mainly originate from a plant, tofu hotdogs are still highly processed foods.

The Organic Delivery Company[60] sells hand-made tofu by Neil McLennan of Clean Bean who takes great care and uses the traditional techniques (2000 years old) to yield a tofu that is incredibly fresh and has a delicate flavor. They also offer a discount when you buy vegetable boxes for high juicing needs (Gerson therapy).

<u>Nuts and seeds</u>

These are fantastic foods, full of nutrients and good fat. Ideally you would eat them in their raw form rather than roasted in oil and then rolled in salt. Experiment with soaking them as it changes the texture. I like soaking almonds in water in the fridge as it makes them a bit buttery which is delicious in porridge or chopped and sprinkled over salads or stir-fried vegetables. Nuts provide protein as well as fat so they help slow down the release of sugars in fruits which is helpful if you tend to 'crash' eating fruit on its own.

Also if you need to put on weight, make 'nutshakes' using rice or almond milk, a banana, a tablespoon of ground flaxseed and a tablespoon of almond butter, cashew butter or any other type you like. For even more bulk, add a scoop of protein powder.

I think all seeds are good for you. I particularly like pumpkin seeds for their high zinc content which is good when healing. Make a mix of different seeds and keep them in the fridge to toss on salads or cereals. Throw a blend together with raisins and keep a little bag in your purse as a snack so you have a healthy option on the run.

---

[60] See Resources - Products

Liquids

Water

Keeping yourself well hydrated is essential for good lymph health, and for skin care and wounds. You need to have sufficient liquid in your body to move the fluids essential to healing.

Make sure you drink enough water, at least 1½ liters per day even if you do not feel thirsty (this is controversial but I call on ten years of clinical experience that most people are chronically dehydrated). If you dislike the taste of plain water, add a squeeze of fresh lemon or lime which contains Vitamin C and supports the liver.

Besides water, which ideally is filtered or distilled, healthy drinks include green tea and red wine *in moderation.*

Green tea

Green tea contains a tremendous amount of antioxidant properties which assist healing.[61] Green tea does contain caffeine so be cautious if you are sensitive and don't drink it after midday. Other herbal teas are fine and dandelion helps support the liver while nettle helps support the kidneys. These teas assist the body by keeping the eliminatory processes working smoothly, which is good when your body is conducting repair work.

---

[61] Qin Y, Wang HW, Karuppanapandian T, Kim W., 2010. Chitosan green tea polyphenol complex as a released control compound for wound healing. *Chinese Journal of Traumatology*, 13(2): 91-5.

Red wine

If you are going to have any alcohol, red wine has redeeming qualities through its antioxidant properties. Remember that we're talking about a small glass a couple of times a week here: not a personal bottle daily. I have spoken with women who say a glass of wine helps them cope with the enormity of the situation and I say that's fine, just be sensible. Try to give yourself more nights off the drink than on, do not drink on an empty stomach and buy organic wines where possible. These are lower in preservatives and therefore less of a burden to the body.

Milk and dairy

Professor Jane Plant, author of *Your Life in Your Hands,* is adamant about fully excluding all dairy products during cancer treatment (and beyond), including yoghurt.[62] Her stance is very firm and she provides excellent evidence for her argument. Her book is most definitely worth reading and then you can make your own decisions about dairy. Indeed in my own research I have come across many studies that link milk with various types of cancer. However no one is completely conclusive so if you cannot bear to stop eating dairy, make some minor changes.

Swap to goat and sheep dairy products as these have been found to be more easily digested than cow's products. The protein and fat molecules are smaller and therefore easier to break down. As always, go organic as there is less drug residue in the finished product. Cheese lovers, grate for flavor rather than eating large hunks of it.

---

[62] Plant, Jane, 2007. *Your Life in Your Hands.* London: Virgin Books

Nutrition

What about your bones? Evidence gathered during the past 20 years indicates that osteoporotic bone fractures are highest in countries that consume the most dairy, calcium and animal protein. There is actually little or no evidence that dairy benefits bones – however there is evidence that consuming dairy may contribute to the risk of prostate and ovarian cancers, autoimmune diseases, and some childhood ailments. [63]

I provide studies that buck our beliefs for two reasons: one is to show you that not even the experts can agree on what we should eat and secondly, we cannot all be crammed into the same box. Furthermore all industries are vying for our attention and money. Advertising is very clever these days. As the song says, "don't believe the hype". The best way to know how to feed yourself is to learn what works for you and what makes you feel strong, vigorous, energetic and above all, nourished.

Believe me you can go round in circles when it comes to nutrition. The main point is to start looking at your diet carefully and see where you can improve. Keep a food diary to associate how you feel with what you eat. Once you connect your food choices with your energy levels and moods you can start to make adjustments so that the majority of your diet fuels you properly and nourishes your every last cell. Consult a qualified Nutritional Therapist if you need guidance.

---

[63] Lanou, AJ, 2009. Should dairy be recommended as part of a healthy vegetarian diet? Counterpoint. *The American Journal of Clinical Nutrition,* 89(5):1638S-1642S.

The best diet to follow while healing is simple, really:

> - Keep everything as close to nature as possible
> - Avoid highly processed foods
> - Eat enough foods with Omega-3 fatty acids
> - Aim for seven to ten servings of fruit and vegetable a day
> - Drink plenty of water
> - Everything else in moderation

I try not to 'ban' foods as this sparks the inner rebel.

Look for healthy alternatives, switch to organic, do more of your own cooking and most importantly, enjoy real food.

Nutrition

Recommended reading

- *Eat to Live* by Joel Fuhrman M.D. (2003, New York: Hachette Book group)

- *Rainbow Green Live-Food Cuisine* by Gabriel Cousens M.D. (2003, California: North Atlantic Books)

- *Your Life in Your Hands* by Prof. Jane Plant (2007, London: Virgin Books)

- *The China Study* by T. Colin Campbell & T.M. Campbell II (2006, Dallas:BenBella Books)

- *Fats that Heal, Fats that Kill* by Udo Erasmus (1986, Canada: Alive Books)

The charts on the next two pages are for reference. Photocopy and keep with the shopping bags as a reminder.

Yes please:

Fruit	All fruit especially berries.
Vegetables	Include plenty of the non-starchy ones. (Asparagus, cabbage, broccoli, carrots, tomato, mushroom, onion, garlic, green beans, cucumber, celery, peppers, courgettes/zucchini, aubergines/eggplant).
Greens	Eat with wild abandon – aim for two servings a day. Add fresh herbs to foods after cooking.
Grains	Whole grains: brown or wild rice, whole grain pasta, rye or spelt bread, porridge.
Pulses	Adzuki, black, butter, chickpea, kidney, navy, lentils, minimally processed tofu.
Fish	Ideally oily fish 2-3x a week, shellfish occasionally.
Eggs	Use organic free range.
Meat	Small amounts of organic – poultry mostly or game. Limit red and fatty meats.
Sweeteners	Soaked dates, maple syrup, honey (Manuka!)
Oils	Cold pressed olive, flax or hempseed oil. Keep in the fridge.
Nuts & Seeds	Ideally eaten raw in salads or porridge or in dips for fruit and vegetable.

Nutrition

Less of these:

Refined sugar	Robs the body of nutrients to break it down, upsets the adrenal glands, and puts weight on around your abdomen.
Large amounts of dairy (milk, butter, cheese, yoghurt)	Possibly linked to increased risk of cancer. Keep portions small and organic, switch to goat and sheep products.
Trans or hydrogenated fats	Lethal!
Fried foods	Full of Trans fats, very hard on the liver.
Coffee	Over stimulates the body – you need to rest and heal.
Alcohol	Avoid or have sparingly – ideally organic red wine.
Tobacco	#1 cause of cancer.
Large portions of red meat (pork, beef, lamb)	Harder on digestive system. Chew thoroughly.
White flour or white rice	Glue paste. Use in children's projects to stick paper together. Similar effect on your innards.

Healing Diet Meal suggestions

Breakfast:

- Include fruit such as strawberries, pears or bananas cut up in porridge, quinoa or amaranth with a sprinkling of seeds.

- Make a nutshake using soy, rice or nut milk and add different fruits (frozen berries too) and ground flaxseed. Add a tablespoon of whey powder (see supplements section) and a spoonful of almond butter if you need more calories.

- Egg and veggie omelet using onion, tomato, peppers, broccoli and spinach with whole grain toast.

- An apple cut into sections or banana smeared with nut or seed butter.

- Whole grain toast with nut butter and sugar free jam or mashed banana or raspberries.

- Whole grain toast with slice of goat or sheep cheese, mashed avocado and a bit of natural sea salt.

- Scrambled eggs with salmon.

Nutrition

Lunch/Dinner:

Always include some type of raw vegetable with each meal. This can be in the form of a side salad, chopped fresh herbs or grated carrot on top. Raw foods contain enzymes that help you break down the food and access the nutrients.

- Beans and rice cooked with onions, garlic, peppers and celery topped with cucumber, avocado, fresh herbs and tomato or mango.

- Vegetable soup (meat or fish used sparingly for flavor) with beans or lentils added for the extra nutrients and fiber.

- Stir fried vegetables with brown rice. Depending on your choices include fish, tofu, pulses or lean meat.

- Whole grain pasta with fish/meat and vegetables.

- Jacket potato with hummus and grated vegetables such as beetroot and carrots.

- Hummus and cut veggies such as celery, carrots, red peppers and cucumbers. Whole grain pita for dipping.

- Large Romaine lettuce leaves can be used as a 'wrap' for various fillings as a way to increase your vegetable and greens intake. Wash and let air dry before using as a wrap.

Pudding:

- Fruit salad is always healthy. Use a variety of fruits and make a dressing of fresh lemon, a touch of honey and cinnamon. Sprinkle on slivered almonds or seeds for extra protein.

- Raw food recipe books have fantastic healthy desserts and creatively blend flavors together – you will forget all about the processed overly-sweet fatty versions once you try these! Raw chocolate is gorgeous and I like the company Booja Booja… a lot!
    - Some raw food or living food websites full of recipes:
        - www.living-foods.com/recipes
        - www.fresh-network.com

Recommended reading:

- *Eat Smart Eat Raw: Detox recipes for a high energy diet* by Kate Wood (2002, London: Grub Street)

- *Living on Live Food* by Alissa Cohen (2005, Cohen publishing)

- *Green for Life* by Victoria Boutenko (2005, Raw Family Publishing)

Nutrition

Super snack:

Green Smoothies are ideal snacks. Blending the whole food retains the nutrients along with the fiber. Make in the morning and sip through the day.

I use a simple hand blender. Chop the larger or tougher vegetables first and add more water if the blades won't turn. Experiment with different types of greens to keep the flavors varied. Here are some of my favorites:

- Whiz a whole pear (minus core), banana and 5 strawberries with a splash of water, squeeze of lime and 3 romaine lettuce leaves or a handful of baby spinach.

- Tomato, cucumber, celery, coriander or basil and watercress with a squeeze of lemon - more savory than sweet.

- Ripe pears, berries and fresh mint

- Cucumber, lamb's lettuce and melon

- Watermelon and mint

Otherwise most of my snacks consist of fruit and nuts or hummus and veggies. There are also many healthy snack bars available now so see what you like. Read the labels for hidden sugars and fats.

Many of my recommended reading selections for the Nutrition section focus on vegetarian diets or raw food diets. These are listed to give fresh insight to the standard western diet. Personally I would say that going 100% raw is not recommended when you are recovering from surgery or undergoing cancer treatment. Increase your vegetable and fruit intake overall and this will automatically raise your nutrition levels.

Please do not be tempted to do any drastic detox diets. You must be in strong health to do these and even then you feel quite horrible while your body cleans. Save it for when you are more robust. By all means add juices and smoothies to a healthy diet and eat from a wide range of foods.

Use the books to get ideas about different ways to prepare food that do not call for the high amounts of fat, sugar and salt most recipe books suggest.

Vegan cookbooks teach you how to convert many favorite recipes without using milk or butter should you choose to eliminate dairy.

Above all else, experiment in the kitchen and see what creations you can make that are healthy and delicious. Have fun!

Supplements

We are exposed to a staggering amount of environmental toxins every day and in order to excrete these from the body we need sufficient amounts of minerals, vitamins, enzymes and co-factors. Additionally when the body is under stress from either disease or surgery, nutritional needs increase dramatically and supplements can assist a good diet.

Dr. Linus Pauling, two-time Nobel Prize winner, said that every sickness, every disease, and every ailment can be traced to a mineral deficiency. Intensive farming has stripped much of the nourishment from our soil. The 1992 Earth Summit Report identified severe mineral depletion of the world's farm and range land soil. If the soil is depleted, the plant is depleted and any animal eating that plant is by default depleted.

Percentage of Mineral Depletion from Soil
During The Past 100 Years:

North America	85%*
South America	76%
Asia	76%
Africa	74%
Europe	72%
Australia	55%

* Some US farms are 100% depleted and some are 60% depleted, the average is 85% depletion as compared to 100 years ago. This is worse

than in any other country in the world because of the extended use of fertilizers and "maximum yield" mass farming methods.[64]

Even eating an extraordinarily healthy diet may not be enough to give you the complete nutrition you need when recovering from surgery. I eat a 95% organic diet and I still take supplements because of living in a city where the pollution is higher. I know that when I stop taking my supplements my energy drops; so I keep taking them.

Let me ask how confused you are when you go to the health store or pharmacy and see rows and rows of different vitamins – it's a thriving business. Which one do you take? Which brand do you choose? Is price a reasonable measure? I am giving you my opinion on how to navigate the hundreds of products available. Regardless of the brand you take, please make sure your supplements are high quality and not full of fillers. If it costs next to nothing there is a good chance it contains next to nothing.

Pre-operative supplementation is definitely indicated for cancer patients. Antioxidant vitamins and minerals, Omega-3 fatty acids and several amino acids are able to modulate inflammation and associated oxidative stress thus maintaining or improving immune function.[65] It is therefore recommended you start a targeted supplementation program as soon as you can.

---

[64] TJClark website http://www.tjclark.com.au/colloidal-minerals-library/soil-depletion.htm

[65] Xu J, Yunshi Z & Li R, 2009. Immunonutrition in surgical patients. *Current Drug Targets*, 10(8):771-7.

Supplements

Foodstate nutrients

Most of the available supplement nutrients are made in isolation; they are chemical salts which are inexpensive to manufacture and have a long shelf life. Rationally it makes sense that taking additional amounts of a certain nutrient will increase levels in our bodies, however the body is programmed to receive nutrition as a package deal in the form of whole foods. Obtaining nutrients in 'food state' makes sense. Dr. Kim Jobst[66] explains how Foodstate nutrients[67] are different to the other vitamins on the shelves.

When Foodstate nutrients are analyzed the structure and function are the same as real food and they are classified as food rather than 'vitamins' by the regulators. Being the same structure as food allows for far better absorption and assimilation of the Foodstate nutrients over chemical vitamins – in some cases quite dramatically so.

The dosage of Foodstate nutrients is low because when the body actually assimilates the nutrients there is no need to take mega-doses in the hopes some of the isolated chemicals get to the cells. Additionally Foodstate formulas contain the special carrier proteins and other substances that allow the body to recognize the nutrient. The complex relationship between our digestion and food simply cannot be reproduced in a lab. For optimal results the body has to receive nutrition in the form of recognizable real food and Foodstate nutrients are just that.

---

[66] See Resources – People
[67] See Resources – Products

Dr. Jobst's recommends supplementation with Foodstate nutrients to his patients as a preventative measure. He gives his suggestions for before surgery, immediately after and then long-term maintenance.

Pre-operative supplementation

Ideally start supplementation with Foodstate nutrients one month prior to surgery or as soon as you are able.

- Multivitamin and Mineral formula
- Vitamin B Complex plus Vitamin C
- Trace minerals
- Antioxidant formula plus CoQ10
- Essential Fatty Acid Complex

Supplements

Immediately after surgery

In addition to the nutrients taken before surgery add extra protein, Bromelain and Vitamin D.

- Soy whey protein: this is 95% soluble and quickly assimilated to provide protein needed for wound healing, tissue regeneration and immune system support.

- Bromelain: this comes from pineapple cores and has a double impact on fighting inflammation.[68] This natural substance is a gentle giant that would benefit any post operative situation.

- Vitamin D3: controls the body's innate immune response, affecting a wound's ability to heal.[69] It also supports mood, helping to prevent depression at a vulnerable time.

---

[68] A study shows that Bromelain has distinct pharmacological promise. Its properties include an interference with the growth of malignant cells, the inhibition of platelet aggregation (clotting), anti-inflammatory action and skin debridement properties (remove dead tissue). Taussig SJ & Batkin S, 1988. Bromelain, the enzyme complex of pineapple (Ananas comosus) and its clinical application. An update. *Journal of Ethnopharmacology*, 22(2):191-203.

[69] Richard L. Gallo, M.D., Ph.D., professor of medicine and chief of UCSD's Division of Dermatology and the Dermatology section of the Veterans Affairs San Diego Healthcare System, says "Our study (appearing online in advance of publication in the March 2007 issue of the *Journal of Clinical Investigation*) shows that skin wounds need vitamin D3 to protect against infection and begin the normal repair process. A deficiency in active D3 may compromise the body's innate immune system which works to resist infection, making a patient more vulnerable to microbes."

Long term supplementation

To stay in optimal health it is advisable to continue supplementation given the status of the soil and our general environmental toxicity exposure.

Remember though - food first: get your diet in top form, and add in the extra support to keep you in the best health possible.

Take the following on a daily basis:
- Probiotic (multi-strain) formula[70]
- Vitamin D3
- Vitamin B Complex plus Vitamin C
- Antioxidant formula plus CoQ10
- Multivitamin and mineral formula
- Essential fatty acid complex

Dr. Jobst recommends an annual test for dysbiosis (microbial imbalance in the body) through a stool test or gut fermentation test. Genova Diagnostics Laboratories provides these tests. It is always advisable to have your GP, nutritional therapist or other qualified healthcare provider go through the results with you.

---

[70] If avoiding dairy use a dairy-free probiotic supplementation to maintain intestinal balance with beneficial bowel flora.

Extra dietary support

Nature's Living Superfood
This a powdered, mineral rich combination of various 'superfoods', packed with antioxidants, chlorophyll and tens of thousands of invaluable phytonutrients. The formula includes:

- **Land vegetables**: whole leaf barley grass, whole leaf wheat grass, nettle leaf, shave grass (horsetail), alfalfa leaf juice, dandelion leaf juice, kamut grass juice, barley grass juice, oat grass juice, burdock root, broccoli juice, kale juice, spinach juice, parsley juice, carob, ginger root, nopal cactus and amla berry.
    - Cereal grasses are very high in nutrition, particularly Beta-carotene, Vitamin K, Folic acid, Calcium, Iron, Vitamin C and many of the B vitamins.
- **Algaes** including spirulina and chlorella, aquatic vegetables Icelandic kelp and Nova Scotia dulse,
- **Enzymes** including mylase, lipase, protease, cellulase, Bromelain and papain
- Comprehensive **probiotic mixture** of beneficial organisms.

Start with ½ tsp daily in juice or water and increase to one or more heaped teaspoons. You can find this product online through various sources or in larger health food stores.

Aloe Vera

Aloe vera is an ancient remedy use to speed healing and is most often used topically. Aloe vera cream reduces post-operative pain and significantly increases wound healing when compared to placebo;[71] whole leaf aloe vera juice facilitates the healing process and inhibits microbial growth with no side effects.[72] While the topical application of aloe is well known, research indicates that aloe vera juice taken internally also helps heal external wounds.[73]

I like Pukka Herbs[74] minimally processed 100% organic aloe vera juice. Pukka's aloe vera only contains the inner leaf gel which has the highest concentration of the active healing ingredients. Furthermore their juice does not contain synthetic preservatives such as potassium sorbate, ascorbic acid or sodium benzoate. It is preserved in just 0.1% of citric acid made from tapioca. Take as directed.

---

[71] Eshghi F, Hosseinimehr SJ, Rahmani N, Khademloo M, Norozi MS, Hojati O, 2010. Effects of Aloe vera cream on posthemorrhoidectomy pain and wound healing: results of a randomized, blind, placebo-control study. *Journal of Alternative and Complementary Medicine*, 16(6):647-50.

[72] Jia Y, Zhao G, Jia J, 2008. Preliminary evaluation: the effects of Aloe ferox Miller and Aloe arborescens Miller on wound healing. *Journal of Ethnopharmacology*, 120(2):181-9.

[73] Feily A, Namazi MR, 2009. Aloe vera in dermatology: a brief review. *Giornale italiano di dermatologica e venereologia*, 144(1):85-91.

[74] See Resources – Products

Supplements

Diet and Cancer: Clinically summarized

> It has been **estimated that 30-40% of all kinds of cancer can be prevented with a healthy lifestyle and dietary measures**.
>
> Low fiber intake, consumption of red meat and an imbalance of Omega-3 and Omega-6 fats may increase the risk of cancer.
>
> On the other hand, the consumption of lots of **fruit and vegetables may lower the risk of cancer**.
>
> Protective elements in a cancer-preventive diet include: selenium, folic acid, vitamin B12, vitamin D, chlorophyll and antioxidants such as carotenoids (alpha-carotene, beta-carotene, lycopene, lutein, cryptoxanthin).
>
> A supplementary use of oral digestive enzymes and probiotics is also an anticancer dietary measure.
>
> A diet drawn up according to the proposed guidelines could decrease the incidence of breast, colon-rectal, prostate and bronchogenic cancer.[75]

You have a good idea of how to take care of your body physically with nutrition, exercise and massage. Now, let's take a look at the energy healing.

---

[75] Divisi D, Di Tommaso S, Salvemini S, Garramone M, Crisci R, 2006. Diet and cancer. *Acta bio-medica: Atenei Parmensis.* 77(2):118-23.

Homeopathy

Homeopathic remedies help support the body's natural and inherent healing system. I have used homeopathic remedies with patients undergoing chemotherapy for the past eight years.[76] Please advise your doctor if you use homeopathy alongside your orthodox treatment.

As much as we cannot physically hold an x-ray or radio wave, we cannot yet fully explain the energetic power of homeopathy. In my clinical experience I have found most people report a positive result when using remedies as an additional aid to healing. The remedies suggested here are more specific to surgery, wound healing and scar support and are not individualized. If you are unsure about taking the remedies without the guidance of a professional please contact a qualified homeopath to help you.

Take your remedies by putting one or two pills under your tongue and let them melt. Take the remedies away from food, drink and toothpaste so you have a 'clean' mouth that can easily relay the message from the remedy to the body.

---

[76] Use of homeopathic remedies in a 12c potency or higher alongside chemotherapy is approved by the Pharmacy department and the Director of Clinical Studies at London Bridge Hospital and this is my guideline here. Remedies in a potency of 12c or higher ensures there is no traceable amount of the raw extract left thereby eliminating the potential for drug reaction with medication.

Homeopathy

Use 30c potency and take the remedy once a day unless otherwise instructed by a professional. If this seems too strong (you are experiencing symptoms that are new or unfamiliar) phone one of the homeopathic pharmacies listed in Resources and ask for 12c or 15c potency and start at the lower potency. A limited range of Homeopathic remedies can be found in larger standard pharmacies and health stores. Contact a homeopathic pharmacy for the more specific remedies.[77]

Pre-op remedies:

Use **CALENDULA 30c** once a day for a week before surgery and for as long as needed afterwards (until the wound is fully healed) as this helps support the immune system and skin.

Use **IGNATIA 30c** or **ACONITE 30c** if needed for emotional support – these are explained on the next page.

Do not use Arnica before surgery as it has blood thinning properties. Arnica is the remedy most people are familiar with and it is brilliant post-operatively but you do not want to take it before surgery, ever. People who are on blood-thinning medication should avoid Arnica altogether.

---

[77] See Resources – Products

> **For emotional support:**[78]
>
> **IGNATIA 30c** taken as needed up to six times a day to help with feelings of helplessness or intense emotional outbursts. This is one of homeopathy's premier grief remedies and is useful when grieving a loss of any kind whether physical, mental or emotional.
>
> **ACONITE 30c** is an excellent remedy that can help with fear, anticipation and panic attacks. Use up to six times a day.
>
> Another good post-op remedy is **STAPHYSAGRIA 30c** if you feel angry, humiliated or invaded after the surgery. Usually only a couple of doses are needed to help clear the energy.

> **Immediately after surgery:**
>
> Now use the **ARNICA 30c** or even more specific use **BELLIS PERENNIS 30c** which is very similar to Arnica but has an affinity with the torso of the body. Take three times a day for one week to help with trauma to the soft tissues.
>
> If you are feeling very spaced out or sick after the anesthetic take three doses of **PHOSPHORUS 30c** in one day to help you ground yourself again.

---

[78] If you are experiencing depression, pain or complications from your surgery you must speak to your Consultant first and then seek a qualified homeopath. These remedies are to help you through the initial stages of surgery and recovery. Anything more complicated requires a full professional consultation.

For scars:

Try and find these remedies in a lower potency, either 12c or 15c and take once a day for a month. The lower potency is more resonate with the physical body. If all you can find is a 30c that is still very useful. After a month, stop taking the remedy for a week to evaluate your scar. If it keeps its shape and the area around it is soft and pliable you may not need the remedy any longer. If the area tightens up again, carry on with the remedy for another month and re-test.

THYOSINIMINUM 30c (thy-os-ini-my-num) may help prevent scar adhesions and restrictions. Established, solid scars may smooth out with this remedy as it helps with skin elasticity.

The second remedy that can help with scars is **SILICA 30c** which is especially good if the scars are painful to touch, become thickened into keloids or are nodular. These scars may also be slow to heal and the patient may feel very shy or withdrawn after surgery.

The third suggestion is **GRAPHITES 30c**. This remedy may help if the scar is hard or has a burning or tearing pain associated with it.

> **For healing:**
>
> **CALENDULA 30c** twice a day is wonderful for supporting overall healing, especially if your scar is not mending well. Use this remedy internally while also using Calendula cream or oil topically on the scar for double benefits. Carry on for as long as necessary.

> **For lymph:**
>
> **SCROPHULARIA 30c** taken once a day for a month can help support the lymphatic system.

> **For liver support**:
>
> Use **CARDUUS MARIANUS 30c** once a day after surgery for a month or longer if feeling sluggish, experiencing constipation or general 'blahs'. (Consult your doctor immediately if you have a yellowish tinge to the eyes or skin.)

As mentioned previously, if you are unsure about taking these remedies, find a qualified Homeopath to help you. These are generalized recommendations based on my clinical experience.

Bach Flower Remedies

Ranjni Janda[79] discusses different Bach Flower Remedies most often used for emotional support while healing. They can be used alongside any type of treatment. There are 38 remedies in all and these are Ranjni's top choices for those recovering from breast cancer surgery or undergoing chemotherapy.

- **Crab apple**: unhappy with appearance, have difficulty adjusting; feel ashamed or embarrassed about self. Also excellent for any skin condition that makes the person feel 'less than' such as eczema, acne, all wounds and scars.

- **Gentian**: can't go on. Feel apathetic because nothing has worked.

- **Elm**: overwhelmed by responsibility

- **Agrimony**: hides problems behind a cheerful face

- **Centaury**: easily led, quiet, gets on with it, don't like making a fuss, hate confrontation

- **Cherry plum**: very anxious, almost on the verge of a breakdown

- **Oak**: exhausted, trouble carrying on, reliable yet overly tired

---

[79] Registered Homeopath, Acupuncturist and Bach Flower practitioner

- **Wild rose**: resigned, don't see a possible recovery, don't try to improve, hopeless

- **Olive**: excellent with chemo – lack of energy, exhausted in body and mind after illness

- **Pine**: apologize for being ill

- **Willow**: self pity and resentment

- **Mimulus**: fear of known things like illness, pain, death

- **Larch**: lack of confidence

- **Walnut**: protection from change and outside influences

- **White chestnut**: stress, stuck on same unwanted thought, obsessive, worrying thoughts that are impossible to control

- **Rescue Remedy**: This is a widely known combination that is sold in many larger chemists already. It is for times of acute stress and has a combination of Rock rose, Impatiens, Star of Bethlehem, Cherry Plum and Clematis. It is the remedy to be used in emergencies or if facing a stressful event.

Bach Flower Remedies

To administer Bach Flower Remedies, take straight from the bottle, four drops on the tongue four times a day. If you are taking a combination of remedies, use up to seven and mix together in a stock bottle. You can either take four drops of this combination as described above or put two drops into a bottle of water to sip through the day.

Nelsons Homeopathic Pharmacy[80] sells complete kits of all 38 Bach Flower Remedies or you can buy a selection of the individual remedies and mix them yourself.

Another useful website for Bach Flower Remedies is www.bachfloweressences.co.uk which has 'The Remedy Chooser' to help you put together a blend.

---

[80] See Resources – Products

Metaphysical Healing

You are more than the body you walk around in. You are more than your dress size, you are more than your cancer and you are far more than your scar. You may identify yourself through things, places or other people's opinions. You may look for outer confirmation to tell you that you're okay, you're acceptable, and that you are enough. Many women constantly judge themselves harshly: something is wrong, horrible, ugly, out of place, unacceptable. And now with this scar...

Shhh.

Go in. Turn inwards and listen for the still voice inside. Let this be your guide. You will find such courage and strength available to you – all you have to do is go in and discover your own inner truth. I will give you various tools to help you release some of the pain you carry and to free yourself from heavy emotions. You will feel lighter and brighter with each release and as a result you can find peace.

Metaphysical Healing

"And a woman spoke, saying, Tell us of Pain. And he said:

Your pain is the breaking of the shell that encloses your understanding.

Even as the stone of the fruit must break, that its heart may stand in the sun, so must you know pain.

And could you keep your heart in wonder at the daily miracles of your life, your pain would not seem less wondrous than your joy;

And you would accept the seasons of your heart, even as you have always accepted the seasons that pass over your fields.

And you would watch with serenity through the winters of your grief.

Much of your pain is self-chosen.

It is the bitter potion by which the physician within you heals your sick self.

Therefore trust the physician, and drink his remedy in silence and tranquility:

For his hand, though heavy and hard, is guided by the tender hand of the Unseen,

And the cup he brings, though it burn your lips, has been fashioned of the clay which the Potter has moistened with His own sacred tears."

~Kahlil Gibran from *The Prophet*

Burning Letters

I give this exercise to my patients on a regular basis. We have so many stored memories in us, many unpleasant, and we can be easily triggered over and over. A wounding word from someone decades ago can still cause a reaction today. Have you ever found your adult self reacting to something as though you were a child? Do you ever stop and wonder where on earth it's coming from?

Sometimes we're upset with people from our present or past and we don't know how to talk about it because we just aren't sure what is really wrong. So we swallow it until the next time those feelings are triggered and we find ourselves back in the same old argument where no one is listening or moving forward.

Writing and then burning letters allows you to 'speak your mind' freely and safely. No one else is to see these letters. You can explore the depth of your emotions and let loose on the page. Your letters are addressed to anyone or anything that creates negative energy or stirs those emotions simmering just below the surface. It may be grief, anger, anxiety, regret or guilt. Anything at all that is holding you back from feeling peaceful and happy can be released in this exercise.

It is very easy. You write a letter telling the person or thing how you feel. Pour out the intensity and just let rip. Take as long as you need, write for as long as it takes for you to feel as though you have fully said everything you need to say and then destroy the letter. Do not leave it lying around where it may accidentally be discovered. This must be a private experience for you and you alone.

When you have finished writing, take the letter outside and burn it. All that pain, all the energy tied up in the pain, all the energy of holding it inside, keeping it hidden, is all now released and gone. Let it vanish from the earth and vanish from your life.

You may need to write to the same person several times as more memories or emotions come to the surface to be released and healed. Keep writing and keep burning. In time you will find those old sore spots are gone. Someone will make a comment that two months ago would have set your teeth on edge and now you barely register it. I promise you, this is very powerful work.

Recommended reading:

- *The Dark Side of the Light Chasers* by Debbie Ford (1998, London: Hodder & Stoughton)

- *Women, Food and God* by Geneen Roth (2010: London: Simon & Schuster UK Ltd) – This book is included for those who turn to food for comfort and eat rather than address the emotions. While eating might make you temporarily feel better it will not release trapped emotions and they will keep coming back until you address them. Face the pain and let it go.

Healing Visualization

A healing visualization is more than a meditation. You actively create a scene for your brain to work with which is helpful if you find emptying your mind a challenge. Do this as often as you like. It can be particularly beneficial to do before scar massage. Read through it the first couple of times so you have an idea of where you're going.

Turn off the phone, put a do not disturb note on the door and turn your attention inside. Sit or lie down, close your eyes and relax. Take five long slow deep breaths, and on the exhalation audibly let out a big long sigh. Feel your body melting into softness.

Close your eyes and let your eyes slightly drift upwards as though you are looking at the inside of your forehead. In your mind's eye or imagination, visualize yourself in a beautiful natural setting. Turn around slowly taking it all in.

Ahead you will see a path of soft golden light. Walk down the path until you see a garden. This is your garden. Are there flowers, trees, birds or butterflies? Do you see animals, fountains or buildings? Walk through your garden enjoying the sights, sounds and smells. Take your time.

A short distance away you see a waterfall and a river stretching away to the horizon. Walk to it and find a comfortable place to sit. As you relax, scan your body. Are you holding stress or negative emotions anywhere? Sense your body; ask it to show you where you are tense. When you find the tension or emotion give it a color - whichever instinctively feels right.

Metaphysical Healing

Focus on the tension and the color and once it is clear in your mind, walk over to the waterfall.

The waterfall starts high above, tumbling down into a pool and flowing out along the river stretching beyond your sight. The water is flowing at whatever speed you wish. There is a ledge where you can comfortably sit or stand under the water. Go there now.

Feel the water run over your head, your skin and down your body. It is the perfect temperature. See your body being washed and refreshed with the water. Now visualize white light merging with the water, pouring into your body through the top of your head, filling every cell with pure white healing light and flowing out the bottom of your feet down the river and away. You are like a straw in the middle of the water and the light; it pours right through you.

Focus again on the tension and associated color. Watch as the water pours into that place. See and feel the emotion and color start to fade out and run down your legs and out of your feet, carried away in the river flowing away from you where it can do no harm ever again.

Stay under the waterfall until the color is completely gone, washed away, and pure white healing light is flowing unrestricted from the top of your head out the bottom of your feet, bathing each cell fully and completely. Take your time to wash out all traces of the color.

When you feel the color is gone, plug up the bottoms of your feet. See the white healing light start to fill your feet, your legs, swirl around your knees up to your hips. See the light fill the bowl of your hips and bathe your inner organs; your uterus, ovaries, large intestine, bladder and liver are washed and infused in light. The water goes higher and into your kidneys, into your spleen, pancreas, small intestine, into your lungs, filling your heart with pure white light, ever reaching higher.

The light reaches the top of your torso and spills into your arms, filling your fingers, wrists, elbows and shoulders. It moves up your neck, your face, behind your eyes, all the way to the top of your head.

When the light reaches the top of your head it sprays out of the top of your head like a whale spout. See it filling an oval shape that surrounds your body extending out about two feet in every direction.

See the light filling the shape around you. You are full of pure white healing light. The energy field surrounding and protecting you is full of pure white healing light.

Give thanks to the healing light and return to your comfortable seat. There you will find a gift waiting for you. Ask in your mind what the gift represents. Wait for your inner voice to answer and when you understand, give thanks and place the gift in your heart center.

Finally visualize a symbol of love and ask that it goes to the place in your body where the color or tension used to be. Spend as much time as you need to, letting love soak into that part of you calling for it. To close your meditation, walk out of your garden, back along the path of golden light to the beautiful nature spot where you started.

Take some deep breaths and start to come back to your body. Wiggle your fingers and toes, have a stretch and gently open your eyes. It is useful to journal your experiences and it is best to write just after meditating when it is fresh in your mind.

Chakra Healing

The breasts lie in the region of the body known as the heart center or the Fourth Chakra based on the ancient belief that we have seven main energy centers or chakras in the body running along the spine from the base to just above the head. The color for the heart center is usually depicted as green but also has **pink and gold** connected with it.[81] The associated gland is the thymus which regulates growth and controls the lymphatic system as well as strengthening and stimulating the immune system.

As this book is about breast scars it means that the love center needs extra attention. This can be such a challenge: self-love and self-care are difficult to do if you feel you do not deserve it. If this resonates with you, work on the heart center using gemstones, color and sound therapy as well as aromatherapy. Using these different tools will help remind you to take care of yourself and your wounded parts.

The gemstone associated with the heart chakra is Rose Quartz. The soft pink stone encourages love, tenderness and gentleness and helps you accept yourself, just as you are today. You can wear rose quartz as jewelry or carry a piece in your pocket.

Sound therapy for the heart center is in the note F. The sound is 'ah' as in saying "Ah! I get it!" It is the sound of breaking through, of

---

[81] For the purposes of this book the color pink is more appropriate for the heart center as green should not be used when the energy of cancer has been present. Charles Paul Curcio, Delphi University, Healing with Colour & Sound. www.delphiu.com

understanding and with it there is a sense of joy in the discovery. You can chant 'AH' in the tone of F to activate the heart chakra. You may find your voice cracks initially as you tune to the right vibration. Keep singing. As may be expected the smell linked with the heart is rose. Use a drop of rose essential oil as perfume or mist yourself in rosewater.

All yearning for deep intimate contact, harmony, oneness and unconditional love comes through this chakra. When this chakra is open and balanced we have a deeper sense of purpose, accepting that all the feelings and expressions of life come from a place of love.

Repeated disappointments in love, life or relationships can make it difficult to open up for fear of rejection. We withdraw into ourselves and close down the heart to avoid further pain but in doing so we also shut down the ability to receive love. We become prisoners to our own pain.

Dr. Bernie Siegel[82] illustrates this so eloquently in his wonderful book *Love, Medicine and Miracles:*

> "The miracles come from within. You are not that unloved child anymore. You can be reborn, rejecting the old messages and their consequent diseases. When you choose to love you will have those days when you're not all you'd like to be, but you can learn to forgive yourself. You can't change your shortcomings until you accept yourself despite them. I emphasize this because many people, especially those at high risk of cancer, are prone to forgive others and crucify themselves. I see all of us as being perfectly imperfect, and ask that we accept ourselves that way."

But what happens when the heart is not filled with soft, sweet fluffiness? What if you are furious, angry at your illness and feel forsaken? How can

---

[82] Seigel, Bernie, 1986. *Love, medicine and Miracles*, London: Arrow Books

Metaphysical Healing

you pretend it's all okay when clearly it is not? Marianne Williamson[83] explains that getting the energy up and out of the body is critical to healing and letting the love in. Getting the anger out is part of the process of relinquishing it. She says "the last thing you want to do – ever – is to buy into the insidious delusion that spiritual lives and spiritual relationships are always quiet, or always blissful."

I agree with her 100% and you have to get in touch with that anger to let it go. And yes, nice girls get ticked off too and it's perfectly fine to do so. Acknowledge your buried anger because ignoring it will not make it go away. Face it with the letter burning, use the healing visualization, and use the power of your voice to break open that burning knot inside. Get it out so you can then let the love in fully.

You must live from the heart and trust what is there. Do what makes you happy. Live your life for you first. Spend time with people you love, listen to music you love, hang or paint pictures you love, animals, places, books, movies, food, art – whatever you love, relish in it. Listen to your heart first and follow its messages. You will not be led astray.

Fall in love with your life and your whole self: scars and all.

---

[83] Williamson, Marianne, 1996. *A Return to Love*. London: Thorsons

Conclusion

Keep this book as a companion on your journey to dip in and out of while moving on with your life. As you grow and change so will your needs. Stay with your healing process and make adjustments along the way.

Remember that guilt has no place in self-care.

If you feel you do not deserve the time to take care of yourself then you must look deeper to find out why. If no answers are forthcoming please see a homeopath, counselor or spiritual advisor to help you.

Unconditional love is something most of us crave deep in our souls. We look outside ourselves to find it and are hurt or disappointed when it does not come. Start by giving it to yourself and see what flows from there. I wish you great love and courage on your healing journey.

Adrianna

Contact Adrianna

If you would like to contact me please see my main website for the most up to date details:

www.homeopath.moonfruit.com

or

www.LoveYourScar.com

At the time of printing my contact work number is 0845 230 0474 and the direct dial number is 44 (0)208 942 0507.

My email is Adrianna.Holman@hotmail.co.uk

I welcome your comments and feedback as you help me learn and grow.

Resources

People

Scar Massage Therapists

Amanda Berlyn *Dip. Clinical Aromatherapy, Dip. Remedial Massage, Reiki II.*
Member of the International Federation of Aromatherapists.
Tel: 07957 408 133
Email: Amanda@amandaberlyn.com

Annette Dawson *MAR M.IHAF AC Recognized TATh M.Embody.*
Full member Association of Reflexologists
Tel: 07939 578 701
Email: Annette.dawson1@btinternet.com
Website: www.bromleytherapies.co.uk

Integrated Medicine Physician

Dr. Kim A. Jobst MA(Oxon). DM. MRCP. MFHom. Dip.Ac.
Functional Shift Consulting

Tel: +44 (0)1432 818 090
Email: admin@functionalshift.com
Website: www.functionalshift.com

Breast Consultants

Mr. Nicolas Beechey-Newman MB. BS. BSc. MS. FRCS.(Eng)
Consultant Surgeon and Clinical Director

The Harley Street Breast Clinic
Tel: 0207 908 6071
Email: THSBC.Secretary@unilabs.com
Website: www.theharleystreetbreastclinic.co.uk

The London Bridge Hospital
Tel: 0207 234 2339
Email: Tracy.Dullaway@hcahealthcare.co.uk
Website: www.breastcliniclondon.com

Dr. Mark Harries MA PhD FRCP
Consultant Medical Oncologist
The London Bridge Hospital, The Harley Street Breast Clinic, Harley Street Cancer Centre, The Sloane Hospital, Guy's & St. Thomas' Hospital
Tel: 0207 234 2002
Email: Michelle.Salton@hcaconsultant.co.uk
Website: www.londonbridgehospital.com

Illustrator
Ali Crossman BA(hons), BWY Dip.
Fine Art: Painting and Ceramics at Camberwell College of Art, British Wheel of Yoga Teacher.
Website: www.vishnushakti.com

Photography
Lisa Noel Greenfield
Website: www.lngphoto.com

Publishing Assistance
Tony Loton / LOTONtech Limited
Email: lotontech-mail2010@yahoo.co.uk
Website: www.lotontech.com/publishing

Products: skin care

Dr.Hauschka
Website: www.drhauschka.co.uk

Inlight Organic Skin Care
Phone: 44 (0) 1326 281 114
Website: www.inlight-online.co.uk

Neal's Yard Remedies
Website: www.nealsyardremedies.com

Nelsons
Telephone: 0207 079 1288
Website: www.nelsonshomeopathy.com

Skin Blossom
Tel: 05600 533 049
Website: www.skinblossom.co.uk

Trilogy
Website: www.trilogyproducts.com

Weleda
Tel: UK contact number 0115 944 8222
Website: www.weleda.com

Products: Homeopathic and Bach Flower Remedies

Nelsons Homeopathic Pharmacy
Telephone Mail order: 0207 079 1288
Website: www.nelsonshomeopathy.com

Helios Homeopathy
Tel: 01892 537 254
Website: www.helios.co.uk

Ainsworths
Tel: 01883 340 332
Website: www.ainsworths.com

Resources

Products: Nutritional Supplements

Foodstate nutrients - Nutritional Shift
Tel: 01432 818 090
Website: www.nutritionalshift.com

Pukka Herbs
Tel: 0845 375 1744
Website: www.pukkaherbs.com

Products: Food

Riverford Organic Veg
Buckfastleigh, Devon TQ11 0JU, UK
Tel: 0845 600 2311 / 01803 762059
Website: www.riverford.co.uk

Organic Delivery Company
A156 Nine Elms Lane
New Covent Garden Market
London
SW8 5EE
Tel: 0207 7398181
Website: www.organicdeliverycompany.co.uk

Abel & Cole
16 Waterside Way
Plough Lane
Wimbledon
SW17 0HB
Tel: 0845 262 6262
Website: www.abelandcole.co.uk

Appendix: Different Surgeries

This information is a bit more detailed from the section in the book for therapists or those unfamiliar with the different breast cancer surgeries and what happens during each. There are excellent and comprehensive guides available from many cancer websites and charities.

Lumpectomy

A lumpectomy involves the removal of a tumor or lump and some of the surrounding tissue. It is a form of breast conserving surgery. A lumpectomy can also be called a biopsy, partial mastectomy, re-excision, quandrantectomy or wedge resection.

Mastectomy

A mastectomy is the removal of the whole breast and can be a simple or total mastectomy, modified radical mastectomy, radical mastectomy, partial mastectomy or subcutaneous mastectomy.

- In a **simple or total mastectomy** the breast is removed but the axillary (armpit) lymph nodes remain. No muscle is removed. A 'keyhole' incision results in a smaller scar and is called a skin-sparing simple mastectomy.

- In a **modified radical mastectomy** lymph nodes are removed as well as the entire breast. These are axillary lymph nodes located in the underarm (Levels I and II). This is known as an axillary lymph node dissection. No muscle is removed and the Level III lymph nodes remain. These lymph nodes are above the breast moving at an angle towards the collarbone.

- In a **radical mastectomy**, which is the most extensive type, the surgeon removes the entire breast, Levels I, II and III axillary lymph nodes and also the chest wall muscles under the breast.

There are still some lymph nodes remaining in the area: the supraclavicular lymph nodes just above the collarbone and the internal mammary lymph nodes which are alongside the breastbone. Assisting the remaining lymph nodes will help minimize the risk of lymphedema.

Radical mastectomies are now rarely performed due to the improved effectiveness of modified radical mastectomy which causes fewer traumas to the body.

Reconstructive surgery

Reconstructive surgeries that involve other parts of the body are described next.

- A Latissimus Dorsi (lat flap or Muscle Pedicle Flap) reconstruction uses muscle and skin from the upper back. This is a less invasive procedure, suitable for women with smaller breasts. An oval section of the *latissimus dorsi* muscle is detached along with skin and fat and drawn beneath the skin to the breast area. A breast implant is usually inserted. This method is used particularly when the chest muscles are removed. Scars will be on the breast area, and on the back or under the arm where the flap

Appendix

was taken. One disadvantage is the resultant muscle weakness in the back.

- A relatively new operation suitable for slim women with small breasts is the Free TUG (*transverse upper gracilis*) Flap. This procedure uses tissue from the upper inner thigh, namely the gracilis muscle. This surgery is more suitable for women who do not have much abdominal tissue or do not want abdominal scars. The scar is long and at the top of the leg and there can sometimes be a problem with fluid building up in the wound area on the leg.

- The Gluteal flap reconstructive surgery uses skin and fat, and sometimes muscle, from the upper or lower buttock. This is removed and reattached to create the new breast. It is usually performed when abdominal tissue is unavailable due to previous surgeries or when the woman is very slim. Disadvantages include scarring on the buttock and potential multiple surgeries, both of which will affect wound healing and posture.

    There are two forms of Gluteal Flap breast reconstruction:

    1. The Superior Gluteal Artery Perforator (SGAP) which uses fat and skin from the upper buttock area to create a new breast mound. The gluteal muscle is not cut or moved.

    2. The Inferior Gluteal Artery Perforator (IGAP) Flap. Here, fat and skin from the lower buttock is used to create a new breast mound. No gluteal muscle is cut or

moved; blood vessels are removed with the fat and skin to supply blood to the transplanted tissue.

- In a Pedicle TRAM [84] Flap procedure a muscle is taken from the abdominal area to supply blood to the new breast skin. The procedure uses the body's own fat, usually from the abdominal wall, helping to create a natural feel for the new breast. The *rectus abdominis* muscles are transferred to the chest wall to reconstruct the breast by tunneling under the skin, avoiding the need to cut the blood supply. After this is sutured into place the surgeon performs a reconstruction of the nipple. After the muscle of the abdominal wall has been removed, a mesh is inserted to strengthen the remaining muscle and help minimize hernias or bulges.

- A Free TRAM Flap breast reconstruction uses the same skin and fat as the pedicle TRAM flap, but takes less of the muscle. An entire section of the abdominal tissue is removed and attached to the site of the new breast. Blood vessels are joined directly to the new area resulting in better blood supply as the blood has less far to flow. This method allows surgeons to make a larger breast if required. Mesh may still necessary depending on how much muscle is removed. Massage therapists would be wise to ask if a mesh has been used in the abdominal area before commencing treatment.

---

[84] *transverse rectus abdominus myocutaneous*

Appendix

- A DIEP (deep inferior epigastric perforator) Flap reconstruction is almost identical to a TRAM surgery but no abdominal muscle is taken. This surgery requires extensive training and experience, in addition to special facilities and surgical tools. A high power microscope is needed to reconnect the blood vessels and the sutures used to do this are about the same diameter as a strand of hair.

INLIGHT voucher

INLIGHT Organic Line Softener voucher

Inlight is giving a **30% discount on their Organic Line Softener** dropping the current retail price of £50.60* to £35.42 with this voucher.

Inlight Organic Line Softener will be available from the online store at a 20% discount during Breast Cancer Awareness month (October 2010).

Remember that for every Organic Line Softener sold during October 2010 Inlight will donate £1 to the charity **Yes to Life** and a further 10p will be donated on an ongoing basis with each purchase of the Organic Line Softener.

Please fill out the details on the back of this page, cut out the voucher and send it in to the address below, enclosing a cheque for £35.42 made payable to **Cemon Homeopathics Ltd,** or give them a call with your card details, quoting code Love 30.

INLIGHT at Cemon Homeopathics Ltd, Roskilly's Farm,

Tregellast Barton, St Keverne, Helston, Cornwall, UK, TR12 6NX

t. +44 (0)1326 281 114

info@inlight-online.co.uk

www.inlight-online.co.uk

*subject to price at the time of purchase

Love Your Scar

This voucher entitles you to a 30% discount off INLIGHT's 100% Organic Line Softener.

Name:

Address:

Postcode:

Phone number:

Email address:

Where did you purchase *Love your Scar*?

Circle YES to be added to our mailing list: YES   NO

One purchase available per customer and this voucher is not to be used in conjunction with any other offer.

Soil Association Licence: DJ18427

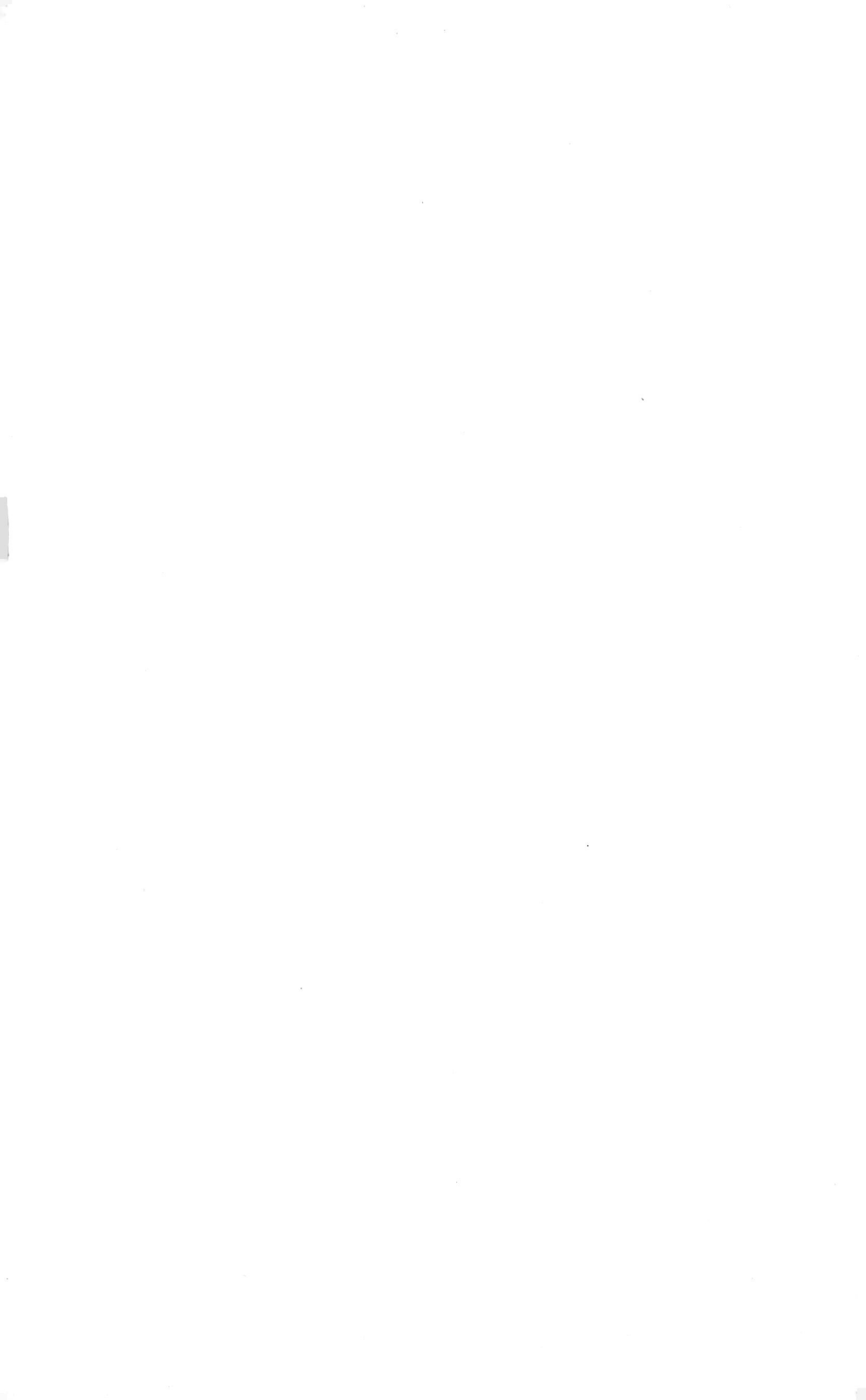

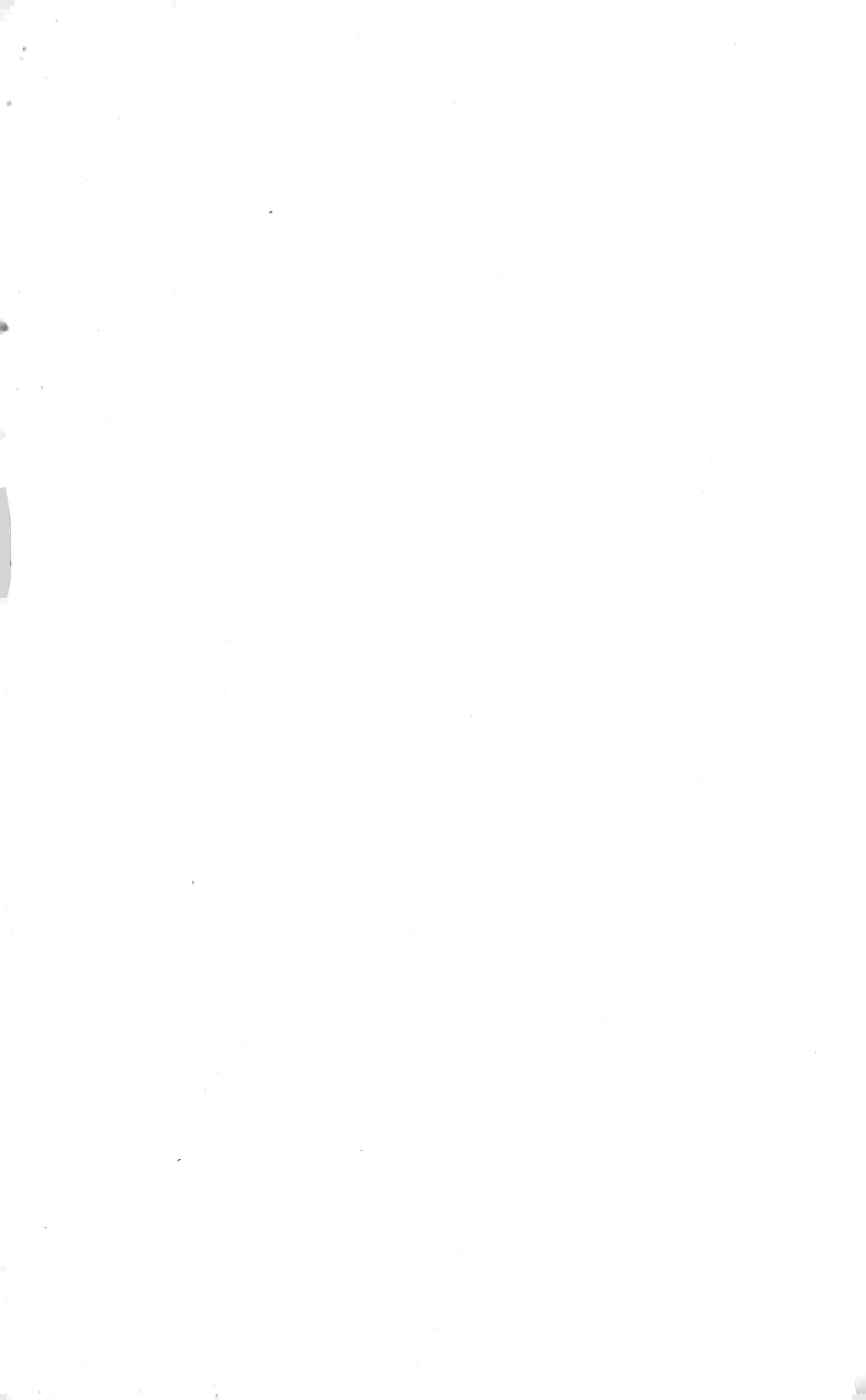